Da Vinci's

BABY BOOMER
Survival Guide

Live, Prosper, and Thrive in Your Retirement

Da Vinci's
BABY BOOMER
Survival Guide
Live, Prosper, and Thrive in Your Retirement

BARBARA ROCKEFELLER & NICK J. TATE

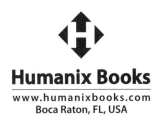

Humanix Books
www.humanixbooks.com
Boca Raton, FL, USA

The DaVinci Guides —
Baby Boomer Survival Guide: Live, Prosper, and Thrive in Your Retirement
© 2014 Humanix Books
All rights reserved

Interior: Ben Davis
Index: Yvette M. Chin

For information, contact:
Humanix Books
P.O. Box 20989
West Palm Beach, FL 33416
USA
www.humanixbooks.com
info@humanixbooks.com

Humanix Books is a division of Humanix Publishing LLC. Its trademark, consisting of the words "Humanix Books" is registered in the US Patent and Trademark Office and in other countries.

Printed in the United States of America and the United Kingdom.

ISBN (Paperback) 978-1-63006-000-8
ISBN (E-book) 978-1-63006-001-5

Library of Congress Control Number 2013948551

Contents

Part II — Considerations for Quality of Life
by Nick J. Tate

Chapter 13 .... **263**
ObamaCare: What Boomers Need to Know

Introduction

THE GOLDEN YEARS OF retirement. For most Americans, they represent the culmination of the American dream of earning a comfortable living, raising a family, and giving back to the community. But for many baby boomers, those golden years are losing their luster.

US Census Bureau statistics show, for instance, that about 10,000 Americans will turn 65 each day over the next two decades. Yet fewer than one in four will have saved enough money for retirement by that age. What that means for many of us is that we are working longer than ever before — well into our 60s and beyond — not because we want to, but because we have to in order to make ends meet.

For those who are able to save enough to retire comfortably, there is another consideration: Federal health statistics show that Americans are living longer than at any other time in history, largely due to major advances in the diagnosis and treatment of many health conditions that once killed people in their 50s and

60s. In terms of longevity, 80 truly is the new 60, with seniors over 85 years of age now the fastest-growing segment of the US population.

But there is also a downside to this decidedly good news: Older Americans are also living with more chronic, costly health problems that accompany them into retirement — cancer, heart, disease, diabetes, Alzheimer's disease, etc. — compared to a generation ago. For nearly one in four seniors on Medicare, out-of-pocket medical expenses exhaust all of their assets and life savings in the final years and months of life.

If these statistics aren't enough to give you pause, consider the following:

- Medicare benefits are unsupportable at current levels and may need to be scaled back significantly to remain solvent, while Social Security taxes will have to be raised if benefits are not cut, something that is politically unacceptable today. Eligibility ages may have to be raised in one or both programs to 67 or even 70, according to experts. When Medicare was created in 1965, 19 million Americans were eligible. Today, it's more than 50 million, and that figure is rising by the day, according to federal Centers for Medicare & Medicaid Services. In 2010, the federal government spent $528 billion to fund the program. By 2020, that spending is projected to hit $1 trillion.

- Seven in ten Americans 65 and older will one day require some form of long-term care in a residential facility, nursing home, adult day-care center, or in their own homes, according to the US Department of Health and Human Services. Yet only one in 12 have actually purchased long-term insurance or arranged for some other means to pay for it.

- Nearly half of Americans 85 and older will develop Alzheimer's disease or dementia and require assisted medical and/or residential care, according to the Alzheimer's Association. In many cases, adult children live in separate cities and are unable to help out with their parents' needs.

In short, these demographic and economic trends add up to a burgeoning crisis of major proportions when it comes to retirement planning for many of the nation's baby boomers. The greying generation that so revered youth and youth-culture is facing the prospect of a bleak future — one that gives a chilling new meaning to Pete Townsend's famous quip: "Hope I die before I get old."

But it doesn't have to be this way. In fact, a little planning and foresight can go a long way toward making sure your hopes and ideals for retirement don't collide with these harsh economic, financial, and health-related realities.

In essence, this is precisely why we've decided to produce this survival guide: to help you navigate your way to a fulfilling, active, and financially-secure future.

What you will learn in this book:

- Smart financial moves you can make now in terms of investment and savings — whether your retirement is months, years, or even decades away — to be sure your golden years are just that

- How to calculate how much you'd likely need to save for retirement based on current US life-expectancy projections and your lifestyle

- Tips for establishing a strong financial profile that will allow you to plan for any eventuality, including a catastrophic illness or unexpected monetary emergency

- What you can reasonably expect to receive in terms of Social Security benefits and other government assistance after you retire

- How to evaluate the best places to live in retirement, based on costs of living, crime, weather, and other quality-of-life factors

- Clear-eyed advice for handling estate planning, inheritances, wills, and trusts

- What the Patient Protection and Affordable Care Act (aka ObamaCare) will mean for you and your healthcare, and how to plan accordingly to take advantage of some new opportunities and minimize the financial risks the new health law may present

- Practical tips for surviving the coming changes and challenges in Medicare, including how to pick a health plan, determining whether you need supplemental insurance, avoiding Medicare- and ObamaCare-related scams, and strategies for maximizing your healthcare dollar

- A guide to choosing long-term insurance, nursing home care, assisted living facilities, and planning for the catastrophe no one sees coming: a serious medical emergency that can deplete your life savings

- A state-by-state list of patient-advocacy agencies and insurance ombudsmen to help with questions and complaints you may have about healthcare providers, insurers, or physicians

- How to craft detailed advance medical directives — including a living will — to make sure your wishes are carried out, should you become incapacitated and unable to speak for yourself

- An age-specific breakdown of recommended health-related screening tests that offer significant protection against cancer, heart disease, diabetes, dementia, Alzheimer's disease, and other conditions

- The latest word from the nation's leading doctors and anti-aging specialists on how boost your health (mentally and physically) and longevity, so that you are not merely surviving in retirement, but *thriving* in your golden years

In short, this book has been written to provide a handy, useful, and practical roadmap to retirement for baby boomers. It was designed specifically to allow you to expand — not limit — your interests, hobbies, social network, community involvement, career pursuits, and your personal goals in retirement.

It's a cliché that all good stories have a happily-ever-after ending. But it is our sincere hope that what you find in this book gives you the wherewithal to make your retirement the richest, most fulfilling chapter in the book of your life — for yourself and your loved ones.

Financial Decisions

Getting Started: Taking Stock

1

THE PHRASE "SURVIVAL GUIDE" in the title of this book suggests ordeals ahead for which you might not be prepared. But while "survival" implies overcoming adversity, this is not your grandpa's retirement. When your grandfather was 60, he was an old man; the baby boomer generation has a younger biological age than chronological age. Maintaining more youthful characteristics for longer is due to healthier life-style choices, better medical care, a cleaner environment, and less hazardous working conditions — more people in offices than digging ditches and working on the railroad.

Accordingly, the average retirement age is rising, too. In the early 1990s it was 57, then by 2003 it rose to 59, and to 61 in 2013. Those nearing retirement say they don't expect to do so until age 67. In many cases, the decision to retire is delayed because of financial insecurity, but for others, retirement is postponed because the boomer is healthy and happy enough in his job to want to keep working.

Moreover, you'll find that most boomers can't imagine what they would do all day if they didn't go to work. Not everyone plays golf. A large minority of boomers who were unhappy with their work are seeking their lifelong, dream career in retirement. Boomers intuitively know that retiring early means dying earlier, too.

Finally, baby boomers are famous for going with the flow — adapting to changing circumstances on the fly. Making it up as you go along, the *ad hoc* style was a hallmark of the 1960s in particular, when social and cultural norms were evolving very rapidly. Aside from goals like completing college or buying a first house, making long-term plans was, for many, too fuddy-duddy. Why go through this effort when conditions will be wildly different in only a few years anyway? Many baby boomers don't know *how* to make a plan. But the fact remains that by the time you are 50, you need to start making a retirement plan if you want to enjoy the same or nearly the same standard of living after retirement.

Retirement offers a chance at re-inventing yourself, perhaps with a dream job or at least a change in lifestyle. Where you live and with whom you spend your time are decisions that require some soul-searching. But whether you decide to retire early, change jobs, or die in harness, the biggest factors are your health and how much money you have or can earn. Not surprisingly, these two factors are not independent of one another. Wealthier people tend to be healthier people, and vice versa. You can be healthy and poor and unhealthy and rich, but on the whole, wealthy people take better care of their health than poorer people, not only because they can afford to, but also because being health conscious is a social norm among the wealthy. Everybody dies, of course, but at what age and under what circumstances does depend, to a great extent, on money.

The connection between health and money is a strong one. In 2013, bankruptcies due to excessive medical bills accounted for three of five bankruptcy filings, affecting 1.7 million people. This is more than bankruptcies due to credit cards or mortgages. Of those in the 45–54 age-group, 170,875 persons filed for bankruptcy because of medical costs, and of those in the 55–64 bracket, 102,080 persons. Those over age 65 who filed for bankruptcy in 2013 numbered 51,719. According to NerdWallet.com, even people (about ten million) with health insurance are accumulating healthcare bills they can't pay off right away, because so many insurance plans feature high deductibles. Some 25 million persons "save" by delaying the renewal of prescriptions or missing doses.

So the paradox is that you need to be healthy to get or stay wealthy, and for many, the cost of healthcare prevents getting and staying healthy.

You are Not Alone

The so-called "baby boomer" generation, defined as those born post-World War II, from 1946 through 1964, number over 76.4 million persons. As US Census data reveals, the bulk of boomer seniors, the fastest-growing demographic in the country, are moving into retirement at an alarming pace. Census statistics for 2012 shows that seniors make up 13.7 percent (43.1 million) of our overall population, compared with 12.4 percent in 2000. The US government estimates seniors will comprise 19 percent of our nation's population by 2030.

Moreover, in addition to the mass numbers, the statistics also show that, as time and economic hardship progress, this group is retiring at a much later age. Those born in 1946 started retiring at age 62 in 2008 and at age 66 in 2012. Today, some 6,000 to 10,000 baby boomers are retiring daily. Companies selling goods and services know it, and accordingly, the range of offerings targeted directly to you is expanding very rapidly (as are the come-ons and scams).

It's likely that viewing the things that worry you from several different directions will water down the fear factor. The act of identifying and naming a worry can, in many instances, go quite far in providing a solution; but to this end, follow-through is in order. It seems that many baby boomers are long overdue for a reality check.

Baby Boomer Worries

What do baby boomers worry about? At the top of the list is outliving one's savings and becoming homeless. Really rich people (the top one percent of the population) don't have this fear; if some calamity should befall their home, they can go to a swanky hotel or just buy another house.

Next on the list is becoming so ill that your insurance doesn't cover medical costs, forcing you to use up all your savings just to stay alive. And still another worry along the lines of illness is falling prey to dementia or Alzheimer's disease. Some research says older people fear losing their marbles more than they fear death.

Third is being cheated — by an insurance company, investment broker, a home improvement contractor, an e-mail scammer, or an unscrupulous relative who finagles your power of attorney and fritters away your savings. According to ConsumerAction.org, those who are 60 and older make up 15 percent of the population, but account for nearly one-third of fraud victims. Advice to avoid being defrauded is available from numerous places, including AARP (AARP.org/money/scams-fraud) and the North American Securities Administrators Association (NASAA.org/2815/nasaa-fraud-center). This topic is covered in more detail in Chapter 7.

Will You Outlive Your Savings?

Chances are the answer is yes.

Life expectancies are rising all the time. If you are 50 today, you will probably live another 30 years. If you are 60, you likely have another 23 years, and if you are 70, another 14 years. Let's say you are 60 to 65 and want to retire to an assisted-living apartment when you are 70. Your monthly income from a pension and Social Security is $3,500, and you have savings of $150,000. An apartment in a first-class, assisted-living facility in your state costs $4,500, and that's before nursing and other specialized care that you might need later on. You would be using your savings ($1,000 per month) for the difference, giving you a maximum of 150 months (12.5 years) with the savings you have.

But your life expectancy is *longer* than 12.5 years. Besides, assisted-living costs will almost certainly be higher by the time you are ready to enter, while your pension and Social Security will go up by only a modest inflation adjustment, if at all. What happens when your savings runs out? You have to move to a less expensive facility — something that is no fun when you're 82. Getting a job at 82 is pretty much off the table. Possible solutions include: (1) starting to save more right now toward your rainy-day fund; (2) buying an annuity or long-term care insurance now against the day your savings run out; or (3) reimagining your plan to include being cared for by a family member (if this is even a possibility).

These are just a couple of the many possible scenarios and a few of the many possible solutions. Perhaps you are among the minority whose situation is different from this one, but for most, these scenarios emphasize the following key points:

- You have only now begun to give consideration to your life expectancy.

- The probability is high that you do not have the financial resources, including savings, to last as long as you will live.

- You need to devise your own plan as soon as possible.

As of March 2013, 57 percent of US workers had less than $25,000 in savings, excluding their homes. This number comes from a survey conducted by the Employee Benefit Research Institute, which also found only 46 percent have a retirement plan and only 14 percent of those in the survey believe they will have enough money in retirement.

In the 2013 EBRI "Retirement Confidence Survey," workers aged 55 and older claimed to have the following in savings:

- 60 percent have less than $100,000 in retirement savings

- 43 percent have saved less than $25,000

- 36 percent have saved less than $10,000

There's a disconnect here. The workers in the survey said they are "confident" they are preparing for retirement properly, but their savings simply do not justify that confidence. The EBRI survey found that 70 percent of all workers surveyed said they believe they are "doing a good job of preparing for retirement," which is true only if they believe they will be getting a hefty defined-contribution pension.

Bottom line: Baby boomers have not been savers.

The following is data collected by the US Census Bureau, which undoubtedly underscores the alarming situation in which both those poised to retire and current retirees find themselves.

This means an ever-rising proportion of baby boomers are continuing to work past 65. The Bureau of Labor Statistics reports that 18.5 percent of those 65 and older were in the labor force in 2012 (24 percent of men and 14 percent of women). Some continue to

TABLE 1-1: RETIREMENT NUMBERS

Average savings of a 50-year-old	$43,797
Total cost for a couple over 65 to pay for medical treatment over a 20 year span	$215,000
Percentage of people ages 30-54 who believe they will not have enough money put away for retirement	80%
Percentage of Americans over 65 who rely completely on Social Security	35%
Percentage of Americans who don't save anything for retirement	36%

Source: http://www.statisticbrain.com/retirement-statistics/ using US Census Bureau data, January 1, 2014

work because they love it and gives them a sense of purpose, but many are working because they must, having failed to save.

An earlier EBRI survey found that the amount of workers currently saving for retirement was 57 percent for those 45 to 54, and 66 percent for those aged 55 and over. In other words, a third to nearly a half of those groups is not saving for retirement at all.

TABLE 1-2: SAVINGS PLUS INVESTMENTS BY AGE GROUP

	Age 45 to 54	Age 55+
Less than $10,000	46%	31%
$10,000 to $99,999	26%	29%
$100,000 to $249,999	12%	18%
$250,00 or more	17%	22%

Source: "2012 Retirement Confidence Survey," Employee Benefit Research Institute and Mathew Greenwald & Associates.

Separately, a Federal Reserve survey found that about 60 percent of both age groups own retirement accounts. Fidelity finds that the average annual contribution is $11,000 to $13,360 for the age group of 45 to 69 in 2013. The Fidelity data is especially informative because it covers 999,000 individuals, an exceptionally large number for any survey.

The Fidelity analysis is broken down as follows:

TABLE 1-3: AVERAGE ANNUAL RETIREMENT CONTRIBUTION

Age 45 to 49	$11,077
Age 50 to 54	$12,880
Age 55 to 59	$13,360
Age 60 to 64	$12,867
Age 65 to 69	$12,505

Source: 2012 Fidelity Investments Analysis of Participants Saving in both a 401(k) and an IRA, http://workplace.fidelity.com/sites/default/files/FF_DC_IRA_032213.pdf

What about home equity? The savings data excludes the value of baby boomers' homes, which can be converted to cash savings either through selling it, re-mortgaging it, or taking out a reverse mortgage. But nationwide, the Federal Reserve reports the median family net worth of those 55 to 64 is $179,400, and those 65 to 74, $206,700, consisting chiefly of real estate. Even if we assume the homes are owned outright (no mortgage or liens of any kind), this is not enough to live on for very long.

How Much Do You Need?

Since the fear of outliving financial resources is the number one concern of baby boomers, and justifiably so, you'll need to do some scenario-building of your own.

How much you need to have saved depends on how long you will live. Life expectancy is a tricky subject and if you do a broad survey of many websites, you will get a broad range of answers.

You can get a life-expectancy estimate using the calculator at Gosset.Wharton.UPenn.edu/mortality/perl/CalcForm.html. The survey asks the usual questions about your height and weight, family medical history, current diet and exercise habits, whether you drive at the speed limit, and so on. The result is your additional life expectancy in years. You can also see how many extra years you will get by changing your behavior in one or more of the categories, like getting more exercise.

According to Social Security's Office of the Chief Actuary, your life expectancy depends on how old you are today. If you are 50 today and are female, your life expectancy is estimated at 85.5 years; however, a 62-year-old woman today has a life expectancy of 86.3 years. A male at 50 today should live to see age 82.3, according to experts; but a man of 62 today has an estimated life expectancy of 83.8 years. As the individual ages, the estimated life expectancy also creeps up — at age 67 his estimated total years are 84.7. (SSA.gov/OACT/population/longevity.html.)

Data gathered by the Census Bureau indicates that the US population of persons aged 90 and above has already been calculated at 1.9 million in 2010, tripling since 1980. In fact, people who are over 90 now constitute 4.7 percent of those over 65. By 2050, the 90-and-over groups will comprise 10 percent of the population.

The Centers for Disease Control and Prevention (CDC), a government agency, publishes life expectancy tables in extreme detail (cdc.gov/nchs/fastats/lifexpec.htm). Data is based on the 2010 census and can be sliced and diced by sex, race, socioeconomic status, education, and numerous other factors for those at birth, and at ages 25, 65, and 75. Overall, life expectancy in the US is about 78.7 years as of 2012, but as always, an average disguises a wide range of possibilities. Yet another interesting calculator can be found at Helpage.org/global-agewatch/about/about-global-agewatch/. You can input your age to find your average life expectancy by sex and country.

Finally, an interesting way to look at life expectancy comes to us from the Internal Revenue Service. The IRS requires minimum distributions from tax-deferred IRA's and some other tax-deferred accounts starting at age 70.5, and calculates the minimums from life expectancy tables. Survivors who inherit tax-deferred accounts get the same treatment. The survivor's life expectancy table is adapted from IRS Form 590. Note that the IRS considers life expectancy at birth to be 82.4 years as of end-2012.

TABLE 1-4: IRS LIFE EXPECTANCY FOR SINGLE SURVIVOR	
Age	Additional Life Expectancy
50	34.2
54	30.5
58	27
62	23.5
66	20.2
70	17.0
74	14.1
78	11.4
82	9.1
86	7.1
90	5.5
94	4.3
97	3.6

Source: IRS Publication 590, http://www.irs.gov/publications/p590/ar02.html#en_US_2013_publink1000231217

The Monster under the Bed: Long-Term Care

So, let's take the case-example in which the baby boomer is 66 today and will live another 20.2 years. Whether this is a financially-comfortable retirement, or one filled with money worries depends entirely on whether his/her Social Security income, pension, and savings combined are sufficient to allow the individual to continue living in his/her own home for the remainder of his/her years. The monster under the bed is deteriorating functionality, even if not accompanied by severe ill-health. Once the boomer needs to rely on home healthcare or leave home for assisted-living or nursing care, the cost of living multiplies exponentially.

The cost of long-term care varies from state to state. With only a few exceptions, long-term care is not covered by any government program, including Medicare/Medicaid. Medicare pays for only about two percent of nursing-facility costs. Medicaid pays for about half, but to become eligible, you have to have dispose of nearly all your personal wealth, as well as jump through hoops, although a large number of states now have a "partnership" program that allows you to keep assets. Medicaid may pay for some assisted-living residences, but most of the cost has to be paid privately. Medicare and Medicaid are primarily healthcare oriented, not housing oriented; therefore, paying for long-term care that is not directly related to health conditions is the responsibility of the individual.

Fortunately, the US Department of Health and Human Services' Administration on Aging has an excellent website that allows you research the costs of different levels of long-term care by state (LongTermCare.gov/costs-how-to-pay/costs-of-care-in-your-state).

The numbers presented on their site are indeed thought-provoking. A retired boomer may be financially secure enough, with sufficient income from Social Security and a pension to live at home alone or as a couple, but add a "homemaker" or home health aide at $32,000 to $57,000 per year, and suddenly the average boomer's savings of less than $100,000 will last only two or three years. You might be better going straight to assisted living, although at the high end, the cost is $72,000/year, or $6,000/month. Baby boomers without savings who are counting on Social Security alone will get an average of about $1,230/month, which implies a lesser facility, to be charitable, if one is even available at that price.

Nursing homes have been around for decades, but assisted living facilities are a relatively new undertaking in the United States. The Assisted Living Federation of America (ALFA), the industry association, was founded only in 1990. As you might expect, the quality of assisted living facilities ranges from awful to the equivalent of a first-class hotel or golf resort. Many assisted living facilities also contain a nursing care facility. You can find information at ALFA.org, (703) 894-1805; AssistedLiving.com, (866) 333-8391; Caring.com, (800) 952-6650; APlaceForMom.com, (866) 344-8005, and many other services that will help you research the field. Another source is CARF.org, or the Commission on Accreditation of Rehabilitation Facilities at (888) 281-6531.

Unfortunately, if you inquire online to get any information at all, you have to give your name, telephone number, and e-mail address, and you know what that means — you will be pestered. Some states have websites that are straightforward, such as Maine.gov, or regional services, like ABCElderCare.net, serving Long Island. As you begin your search, consider whether you have any affiliations that might be useful, such as membership in the Masons (MasoniCare.org, 888-679-9997); or a religious group, like Lutheran Senior Services (LSSLiving.org, 314-446-2475); United Methodist Homes (UMH.org, 877-929-5321); and Catholic Senior Services (CatholicElderCare.org, 612-379-1370). It is likely that these membership affiliations will be cost-effective. Inquiries are free; you should never have to pay someone to find an appropriate senior living arrangement.

Homelessness

Running out of money and becoming homeless is a top fear of people over 65. This is sometimes called "bag lady syndrome." Even rich people have a fear of becoming destitute and living on the streets or skid row, including celebrities (Lily Tomlin and Shirley MacLaine are among those who admit to having bag lady syndrome).

How realistic is the fear? The National Coalition for the Homeless (NationalHomeless.org, 202-462-4822) writes that the number of elderly homeless who go to public shelters is rising nationwide. The demographic research gets a little murky because the main subject is poverty, and while poverty levels are rising in the country, most poverty surveys break down the groups by family composition, not age. Children are counted as children, but the elderly are not counted separately from other adults.

A couple of points do emerge, though. For one thing, mortality rates among the homeless elderly are very high. The combination of failing health and harsh conditions results in a higher proportion of deaths among the homeless elderly (aged 62 and above) than the rest of the homeless population. The demand for low-income housing far outpaces the supply.

The Employee Benefit Research Institute reports that the proportion of older people (65 to 74) living below the poverty line has been growing steadily, from 7.9 percent in 2005 to 9.4 percent in 2009. The latest data from the Census Bureau indicates those over 65 in poverty are 14.8 percent of the population.

It gets worse. For those 75 to 84, the increase in poverty is more pronounced, from 7.6 percent in 2005 to 10.7 percent in 2009. In other words, the older you get, the more likely it is you will fall into poverty. Those 85 and older who became impoverished rose from 4.6 percent to 6 percent by 2009.

The single biggest driver of elderly poverty is medical costs. Not surprisingly, nearly all (96 percent) of the elderly living under the poverty line have a serious health problem, compared to 61.7 percent of the elderly above the poverty line. And 70 percent of those living below the poverty line have suffered critical health problems (cancer, heart attacks, or stroke) compared to 48 percent of those above the poverty line.

Who are among the most impoverished in our nation? Poverty rates for women between 2001 and 2009 were 13 percent, but for men, almost half, at seven percent. Single persons have a higher poverty rate than married couples. Those with less education tend to enter poverty at higher rates than those with higher education. And geography plays into it as well. The Census Bureau reports that nine percent of people age 65 and older lived below the poverty threshold in 2010. But there is a vast amount of geographic diversity in poverty rates, ranging from over 25 percent in Opelousas-Eunice, Louisiana, and Gallup, New Mexico, to less than two percent in Pocatello, Idaho; Helena, Montana; and Ames, Iowa.

Fear of homelessness is understandably justified under two joint conditions: You become ill and the cost of treatment is extremely high, and you have not saved enough to pay for medical expenses. You need not worry about becoming a bag lady or skid-row denizen if you are a millionaire, or if nature smiles on you and you never become expensively ill. And as you probably know, Medicare pays for about 80 percent of medical expenses and for the remainder, you need to have supplementary insurance and/or other long-term care insurance — or lots of savings.

Technically, the probability of becoming homeless and living on the street at an advanced age is not all that high — if you are prepared to accept government aid. Various government programs, including Medicaid, are available to provide housing for the elderly if they are also chronically ill. The problem, of course, is that by the time an elderly person has become homeless, he/she is not materially or psychologically equipped to navigate the corridors of an emergency-housing or nursing-care bureaucracy. Without a phone and an address, homeless people generally (and not just the elderly) get discouraged by the red-tape hurdles.

Provisions of the Affordable Care Act (ObamaCare) are stronger for the truly destitute than for those just above the poverty line. The long-term care portion of the bill was abandoned early in the process, simply because it was too expensive. Like Medicare and Medicaid, ObamaCare targets healthcare costs, not housing costs. Therefore, while becoming homeless is not really likely, the alternative — a Medicaid-funded nursing home — may not be to your liking. Aside from not being able to cope with government bureaucracies, this is one reason why some elderly choose skid row and emergency shelters — the Medicaid nursing home option is too depressing.

The endgame for severe depression is suicide; and it's true that the elderly commit suicide at a disproportionately high rate. According to the American Association of Suicidology (Suicidology.org), in 2010, those over 65 made up 13 percent of the population, but 15.6 percent of suicides, or about 5,994, occurred among those 65 and older in that year.

Older white men commit suicide at a far greater rate than women — 5.25 times more often. White men over 85 had a suicide rate of 47.33 per 100,000, or 2.37 times the current rate for men of all ages (19.94 per 100,000). Actually, the elderly attempt suicide less often than other age groups — but they succeed more often. For all ages combined, there is one successful suicide for every 100 to 200 attempts, or 0.05 to 0.1 percent. But for those over 65, about one in four succeeds. An interesting tidbit is that the rate of suicide by women peaks at ages 45-49, but declines after age 60.

The good news is that elderly suicides are declining from a peak in 1987 of 21.8 per 100,000 people, down 28 percent to 14.9 in 2010. "This is the largest decline in suicides rates among the elderly since the 1930s," according to the American Association of Suicidology.

Baby boomers have failed to save very much, and the lack of savings, combined with rising life expectancies, puts them at risk of being destitute in old age and possibly needing to live in a Medicaid facility that might not meet their standards of comfort. The real culprit: The excessively high cost of medical care is covered only in part by Medicare and supplementary insurance. A basic rule of economics is that increased demand — and baby boomers are demanding more (and more expensive) medical care with every passing day — will bring forth fresh supply under free market conditions, but that can be a lengthy process (e.g., training doctors, building hospitals). No one expects healthcare costs to fall anytime soon, even if the rate of cost-increase levels off.

The Solution

In the meanwhile, the solution is pretty simple — stay healthy enough to avoid an expensive medical emergency . . . and start saving. In fact, save until it hurts, and then save some more.

Dismiss the idea that you are too poor to save. This idea never passes the "So what?" test. You may think you don't make enough to save any money. For this reason, many are apt to say things like, "Even if I could save a dollar a week, so what? At the end of a year, I'd only have a measly $52." And yet at the end of ten years, you'd have $520 plus interest. In practice, you can save a lot more than a dollar a week.

Say your car gets 20 miles per gallon and a gallon of gasoline costs $3.50. Drive 20 miles less per week and put the $3.50 into the savings account. At the end of a year, you have $182 plus interest, and at the end of 10 years, you have $1,820.

Maybe coupon clipping is not your cup of tea, but clip just one coupon per month for a savings of $3.50, and now you are doubling your gas money to $364, or $3,640 after ten years. Join the loyalty or senior citizen discount program at your supermarket pharmacy and any other that offers one, and save another $3.50 per week, tripling your gas money to $546, or $5,460 plus interest after ten years.

If you save the $4 per month ($1 per week) plus the $10.50 from the gas/coupon/loyalty discount, that's a total of $11.50 per week or an average $49.83 per month. Salt a savings account with $10 to begin. Assume an interest rate of 1.5 percent compounded monthly. By the end of ten years, you will have $6,458.64 — not a trivial sum of money.

The calculations can be fun. You can plug your own numbers into an online calculator provided free by the US Securities and Exchange Commission at investor.gov/tools/calculators/compound-interest-calculator. You can also use the calculator by Bankrate.com, pictured here. (Bankrate.com/calculators/savings/simple-savings-calculator.aspx).

FIGURE 1-1: SIMPLE SAVINGS CALCULATOR

Initial Amount:	10.00
Monthly Deposit:	49.83
Annual Interest (Compounded) monthly	1.5
Number of Years:	10

Calculate

Your Result

Your monthly deposit of $49.83 for 10 years with an interest rate of 1.50% compounded Monthly with an initial starting balance of $10.00

Year	Balance
1	$612.24
2	$1,223.57
3	$1,844.14
4	$2,474.08
5	$3,113.54
6	$3,762.65
7	$4,421.57
8	$5,090.44
9	$5,769.41
10	$6,458.64

Final Savings Balance: $6,458.64

Source: BankRate.com, http://www.bankrate.com/calculators/savings/simple-savings-calculator.aspx

And these are the obvious savings opportunities. You can also shop at wholesale clubs, give up dessert at the diner, buy one less cup of coffee per week at Starbucks or Dunkin' Donuts, or borrow books at the library instead of buying paperbacks, and so on. At a guess, you can probably find another $10 per month that you spend on things that you honestly won't miss, or rather, that are worth much less to you than the peace-of-mind of building savings. And when you start feeling put-upon by the savings plan, perhaps add back a consumer item or two. But don't give in to temptation too soon. Give it an honest try for at least a year.

An old joke has it that the robber baron fortunes of tycoons such as J.P. Morgan, Andrew Carnegie, and Henry Flagler came more from compound interest than from railroads, shipping, steel, and oil. If the baron had started with $1 million and added nothing per month, at three percent compounded monthly, in 25 years he would have $2.1 million, more than double the starting balance. Adding $1,000 per month raises the 25-year total to $2.56 million. Another interesting tale is that, when asked to name the greatest invention in human history, Albert Einstein replied "compound interest." This story is probably a myth, but in any case, it makes the point that compound interest is a powerful force.

Here's the rub: You have to take the cash out of your checking account or wallet on the day you make the saving and actually put it in the savings account, either electronically or by physically going to the bank. It's not enough to be proud of yourself for being frugal or a savvy shopper. You have to collect the money, however small the amount, — even $1 per week — at the end of the month, go online or to the bank and make the deposit. The magic of saving and compound interest only works if you make the deposit. You probably know people who are seemingly careful about money yet they never have much and they don't have any savings. You find them at Dunkin' Donuts.

TAKE THE 52-WEEK CHALLENGE:

Starting in the first week of January, put $1 in a piggy bank. Then, for each week, increase your deposit by $1. You may only be saving $10 the first four weeks, but by the last four, you'll be saving $49, $50, $51, and $52. By the end of the year, you'll have $1,378 saved!

Baby boomers need to face what may be some unhappy realities about savings. To begin with, remember the *Rule of 72*. Savings accounts are a necessary beginning to capital accumulation, but in today's low-rate environment, they are simply not sufficient. The *Rule of 72* helps you think about exactly how much money you can get if you opt for the safest investment — a savings account or US government note or bond.

The *Rule of 72* is not 100 percent accurate, because it compounds interest only once a year, but it is a very handy guide when thinking about savings. The rule works two ways:

- Divide 72 by the annual rate of return to find the years needed to double a fixed sum of money, or

- Divide 72 by the number of years you want to save to find the rate of return needed to double your money.

The *Rule of 72* assumes compounding only once at the end of each year, whereas compounding is available nowadays on a daily basis (for large sums), and monthly and quarterly bases. Let's say the current rate is 0.95 percent. How many years will it take to double your money? Divide 72 by 0.95 percent and voila! It will take 75 years to double your money. Alternatively, let's say you will be saving for the next ten years. What is the needed interest rate to double your money? Divide 72 by ten and it will take 7.2 percent to double your money.

The key point is to start thinking about how much you must save and what rate of return you will need to get in order to obtain a truly interesting sum of money at the end. Obviously, current interest rates on savings accounts are not going to do the job if it's going to take 75 years at a rate of 1.5 percent to double your money. And if you were to double your capital stake over 10 years, it will take a rate of return of 7.2 percent, which is not available for no-risk savings accounts today.

To do a thorough review of your possible savings, check out ChooseToSave.org/ballpark/, a division of EBRI. This is an estimator that helps you calculate how much you need to save to fund a comfortable retirement. The virtue of Ballpark is that you can include assumptions about Social Security benefits and other aspects of your financial situation to figure out how much you will have at later ages. The Ballpark estimator is not easy to use because you have to input some information that you either don't know or don't want to guess, such as how long you expect to live and what the rate of inflation will be between now and your retirement date. Still, it will be an eye-opener for some.

Savings accounts are a necessary beginning to capital accumulation, but in today's low-rate environment, it would not be sufficient to boost your wealth or income by any significant amount. This doesn't mean you should not save something at every age. Whether it's two percent or 20 percent or 100 percent of your money management plan, savings are worth having, if only to give you a the peace of mind of a personal safety net.

Chapter 7 covers investments, but even if you are the most savvy of money managers, you still need savings. Remember that after the crash of 1929, it took investors over 25 years to get back to their starting capital.

Calculating the Cost of Retirement

Most people think their expenses will fall after they retire, but surveys show that is not always and universally true, according to Robert Powell, editor of the *Retirement Weekly* newsletter published by MarketWatch.com. Powell, who has been writing about retirement issues for over 20 years, has the judgment to select the best material, and even the letters to Powell are often valuable. He says the conventional wisdom is that you need only about 70 to 80 percent of your pre-retirement income in retirement, and that may be okay as a generalization, but in practice, you may need less in the early years (such as 60 to 65 percent), but need to increase spending in the later retirement years. Necessary spending is not a straight line, but a curve.

Powell reports a Morningstar study that shows the "replacement rate" (i.e., replacing pre-retirement income) after retirement depends on how much you've already saved. If you were saving six percent in a tax-deferred IRA, you'd need 65 percent of your pre-retirement income to maintain your standard of living. If you were saving 12 percent, you would need to replace only 55 percent. There is no one-size-fits-all rule for what replacement income you need.

Logically, you should make a list of things you spend on today — including IRAs and Social Security and Medicare taxes — that will be gone after you retire. And what costs will go up? We need to measure price inflation. The consumer price index for the elderly, dubbed CPI-E, actually goes up by a little more than the general CPI. From December 1982 to December 2012, the CPI-E averaged 3.07 percent, more than 2.92 percent for the general population. This doesn't seem like much, but all factors considered, it adds up to about five percent per annum.

The chief culprit, of course, is healthcare costs, which have been increasing faster than regular inflation. Over the very long period between 1948 and 2012, medical-care costs rose 5.42 percent per year, while general inflation rose 3.63 percent. This works out to a 50 percent higher rate. You may think that a more than 50-year comparison is not warranted, but remember, you are going to have 20 to 30+ years for these costs to affect you. The percentage of your income you will spend on healthcare rises from 5 percent at age 60 to about 15 percent by age 80 — unless you are a low-income household, when the higher healthcare costs are 25 percent of income at age 60 and 35 percent by age 80. To see how the Bureau of Labor Statistics allocates spending between urban households (measured by CPI-U), wage earners (CPI-W), and those over 62 (CPI-E), check out the BLS website at BLS.gov/news.release/cpi.br12396.a06.htm. While four of seven components rose more for CPI-E than for the others, there's no question medical costs are the big inflationary item.

Fortunately and somewhat oddly, starting in mid-2012, healthcare costs stopped rising faster than inflation for other goods and services. As of July 2012, healthcare costs were up only about one percent — the slowest annual inflation rate since the 1960s. The Affordable Care Act doesn't get the credit, since it did not address price levels directly, and instead the change seems to have come from cuts to Medicare, prescription-shopping, and hospitals pulling back a little from outrageous (and abusive) charges.

For your planning purposes, however, it's probably not wise to count on medical-care costs falling. If you are 60 and spending only five percent of your income on healthcare, get ready for that to rise to 15 percent over the next 20 years.

Planning

Some people like to plan their activities in great detail and others like to wing it. When it comes to retirement, planning is definitely called for. Retirement advice and planning has become an industry, complete with advertisers disguising their sales pitches as the new conventional wisdom. You can find numerous sites to guide you, ranging from the banal to the extraordinarily useful. Articles by Joseph F. Coughlin, director of the Massachusetts Institute of Technology's AgeLab, for example, address planning, most of which is of the financial variety, but he also addresses quality of life issues. AgeLab.mit.edu has articles on auto technologies for older adults, as well as robotic technology that helps calm those suffering dementia.

Coughlin asked nearly 200 MIT alumni (average age 79) their top advice for new retirees. Here were their responses:

1. Establish a solid financial plan.

2. Continue to work and expand your interests for as long as possible.

3. Take care of your health.

4. Establish a strong network of friends and family.

Just as "saving" means actually making the deposit in the savings account, the first rule of a solid financial plan is to *write it down*. Financial services provider Franklin Templeton conducted a study demonstrating that 90 percent of people with a written plan made with the assistance of a financial planner are happy with their plan, compared to 44 percent of those without an advisor. This is a somewhat self-serving finding, since people answering questionnaires often want to curry favor with the survey-giver, but it's a remarkable and credible finding.

Advice on how to start a retirement plan can be found from pundits in the general press, certified financial planners, banks, brokers, and insurance companies. Retirement planning is a field boasting information overload. So why do people contemplating retirement find it so hard to seek professional retirement advice? That was the finding of a survey by TIAA-CREF, the pension-fund manager and advisor for schoolteachers and professors. A majority of people know they need advice, but find it hard to obtain and harder still to follow once they get it. About half of the people in the survey said it's "not easy" to find retirement advice. Roughly 40 percent thought retirement advice would cost more than they can afford. And about another 40 percent are taking advice from friends and family — non-professionals. And here's the most arresting item from the survey: Only 25 percent of the respondents who did receive professional retirement advice actually took the recommended actions!

It seems that those thinking about retirement planning are as put off by the advisory industry as those needing a will are put off by lawyers. But retirement planning is too important to leave to chance or advice from friends and relatives (who are probably not qualified). We cover financial planning in Chapter 8.

Bottom line: Seeking retirement advice can be intimidating and overwhelming, causing many to procrastinate when it comes to making a plan. Don't fall into this trap. Rest assured that, with a little tenacity, you can find a qualified professional at an affordable price. In fact, you can't afford not to make a retirement plan!

The following advice will put you on the road to retirement readiness:

DaVINCI DO'S

- If you're just beginning to save for retirement, you should first calculate your life expectancy. If you don't know roughly how long you will be relying on savings, it's impossible to know how much you need to save.

- When researching assisted living options, be sure to consider any organizational affiliations you might have, like Masons or Catholic Services.

- Use the *Rule of 72* in order to calculate the rate of return on savings compounded annually:

  » Divide 72 by the annual rate of return to find the years needed to double a fixed sum of money, or

  » Divide 72 by the number of years you want to save to find the rate of return needed to double your money.

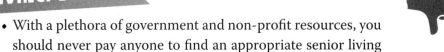

DaVINCI DON'TS

- With a plethora of government and non-profit resources, you should never pay anyone to find an appropriate senior living arrangement.

- Don't think that you don't earn enough to save. Clipping coupons, taking advantage of customer loyalty programs, and foregoing guilty pleasures like a daily Starbucks coffee are all opportunities to start saving. The trick: Make sure that you deposit your savings — even the most meager amount — so that you could start to watch your nest egg grow.

- Don't give up on saving — wait at least a year. By that time, once you see the fruit of your labor, you'll be more motivated than ever to continue.

Retirement Age

2

YOU ARE GOING TO live longer than you ever imagined — a lot longer. Unless you have deeply absorbing hobbies or are wildly rich, you could end up not knowing what to do with all that extra time. Surely you don't want to be an unproductive codger for two or three decades. Boomers will undoubtedly change the way society perceives the elderly and how they see themselves, but it's still a work in progress. You could use the extra time to change careers before retirement, or at least think about a new job after retirement. This is a useful exercise because Social Security is probably not enough to live on, and besides, retiring is, itself, bad for your longevity.

Longevity

You may be surprised to learn how long you should plan on living. For thousands of years, from the Paleolithic era to the Middle Ages, the average life span was 30 to 35 years. From the industrial revolution (roughly 1760 to 1840) to today, longevity has risen by leaps and bounds. The numbers can seem contradictory because "life span" is the expected average from year of birth, while "life expectancy" is a term used to describe both expected life span and the probable remaining number of years you will live based on the age you have already achieved. This is called *life expectancy after attainment of adulthood.*

Michelangelo died in 1564 at the age of 88. Even further back, in medieval times, if you made it to 40, you could possibly make it to 90. This is because you would have already avoided the usual causes of death — accident, plague, war, and infant mortality/death in childbirth. It's not just advances in medical science that get the credit for rising longevity — it's also vast improvement in areas like food safety, sanitation, pollution control, workplace safety, and dozens of other regulatory changes, most of them government-imposed. Today, if you are 60, you can expect to live another 20 to 30 years. For more on longevity, see Chapter 3.

What to Do With Your Extra Years

The baby boom generation poses an unprecedented problem to mankind: what to do with such an abundance of extra years. Mandatory retirement before age 70 was prohibited in 1978 by an amendment to the Age Discrimination in Employment Act for most occupations, but even deferred retirement still gives baby boomers an extra twenty or thirty years — maybe more if research on prolonging life, like telomere repair (units of DNA at the ends of chromosomes that shorten with age), continues to make progress.

It may seem silly to consider an extra twenty years of life "problematic," but it can be. Not only are folks often unaware of exactly when to retire and how to spend their time after they do so, but beyond that, they have difficulty pinpointing their identities in their 70s and 80s. In fact, it's a two-sided problem, because society at large doesn't know how to perceive them either. The social model of a senior — roughly anyone over 70 — as being an old codger is now outmoded, but not replaced by a new model. And in practice, some folks over 70 are codgers, while some folks over 70 are Warren Buffett and Robert Redford, or Barbra Streisand and Martha Stewart. We lack a fresh and relevant prototype.

We are still waiting for a new model to replace the standard set by Robert Butler in *Why Survive? Being Old in America*, first published in 1975 and still in print. It's a grim read, with chapter titles like "No Place to Live" and "Victimization of the Elderly." You probably don't want to run out and buy this book, because despite updates, the author's point of view is unrelentingly negative. "At best, the living old are treated as if they were already dying, and we have not yet emotionally absorbed the fact that medical and public-health advances now make it possible for millions of older people to be reasonably healthy." And our attitudes seem to be in agreement with Butler's take on society's view of the elderly. We pay lip-service to "senior citizens," calling them wise elders, while "seeing age as decay, decrepitude, a disgusting and undignified dependency."

Sociologists study how the elderly are perceived (by nurses, for example) and how the elderly perceive the world (acknowledging that they should no longer drive a car, for instance). Gerontology studies are still fairly basic. Prejudice against old folks, or "ageism", has gotten a fair amount of press attention, since charges of age-related incompetence are often unfair and untrue. On the other hand, some go too far the other way and imagine that the elderly, at least those whose faculties remain sharply intact, enter a state of "gerotranscendence." Whether there is an advanced level of consciousness that is due solely to "elderhood" is debatable.

The term "gerontology" — the study of aging and the aged — was not coined until 1903, although ancient physicians wrote about the medical issues of old age, including forgetfulness. Gerontology is a multi-disciplinary field encompassing social norms and cultural values, as well as biological changes of aging. While the medical science employed to slow biological aging is advancing at warp-speed, psychological aging (sensory perception, cognitive abilities, adaptive capacity, etc.) and social aging have also been getting increased attention since the late 1960s. Social aging has to do with where the older person fits into society. Before the industrial revolution, traditional social norms dictated the elderly's social rank — to be supported by the children and grandchildren in the same house, or more extreme, subjected to senicide (abandoning the elderly to die, as practiced by some groups in

China, Japan, India, and the Inuit culture in times of famine), or somewhere in-between.

In the United States, the baby boomer longevity revolution has yet to resolve the place in society that elders should occupy. Often the elderly enable ageism, or prejudice against the elderly, which stereotypes them as slow-moving, unproductive, and becoming senile. Others resist ageism, often heroically (yet sometimes inappropriately), like 90-year old marathon runners. Resistance also takes the form of humor — everyone loves the cartoon character Maxine, and websites dedicated to "geri-humor" are proliferating (see Everyday-Wisdom.com/senior-humor.html and Facebook.com/geezerplanet).

We are still redefining old age in America. Some people built mother-in-law apartments next to or onto their homes and expect to occupy their own someday, close to their children. Others live a continent away from their parents and want the same thing for themselves — independence and autonomy, even at the cost of a lesser standard of living. Some older folks enjoy being only with people their own age in retirement communities, while others like a mix of ages and enjoy watching children at play. Still others move to Belize or Panama to afford a higher standard of living.

We do not have a social norm in the United States today for how families "should" treat the elderly or how the elderly should treat their grown children. It's not hard to find stories about the baby boomer generation struggling to provide elder care and vowing never to impose the same burden on their own children, and yet everyone has also heard stories of three or more generations living together in harmony. In practice, there never was a golden era in which there was universal consensus on the treatment of the elderly, especially those in ill-health or suffering dementia.

The end result is that the baby boomer generation is in the process of redefining what people face as they retire and become elderly. You need to think about how you want to spend those extra twenty or thirty years so that you are not at a loss when the time comes. And, if you're of average luck, that time will come. The time to start thinking about retirement is before you retire!

Retiring Early Is Dangerous to Your Health

One good reason to think about your life after retirement is that it's not all square-dancing and playing cards. Retirement conjures forth the image of a relaxed lifestyle, including pursuing hobbies that had for so many years been shelved, and not having to deal with coworkers whom you wouldn't ever consider inviting into your home for a cup of tea. In brief: a stress-free existence. Less stress should mean a boost to longevity, right? No. Studies show that the earlier you retire, the sooner you die.

The early retirement/early death phenomenon is more pronounced for men than for women. Death is considered "premature" before age 67, and studies find that one additional year of early retirement causes an increase in the risk of premature death of 2.4 percent, or 1.8 months of life lost. Meanwhile, early retirement has zero effect on female mortality rates. Without intending to stereotype, most women are overjoyed at the fact that they are no longer responsible to work a full-time job and maintain a household, while a man's self-worth is more often tied to his work.

When a man retires his identity in the working-world, depression often sets in, making him more susceptible to deteriorating health. There is also some statistical significance that premature death is higher among those blue-collar males who lost their jobs vs. those who retired voluntarily. However, with a post-retirement plan of attack, men can offset these odds.

Other studies show that workers who retire at age 55 have almost double the mortality risk of those who work into their 60s. In the realm of survival analysis, this is called a hazard ratio. Not surprisingly, low socioeconomic status confers a higher hazard ratio than high socioeconomic status. If you are relatively high up on the socioeconomic scale, retiring early (at 55) carries a 20 percent risk of dying prematurely, whereas if you are in the lower ranks, you have a 60 percent higher mortality risk. The good news is that if you wait until you are 60, you are over the hump. Mortality doesn't change in the first five years after 60 among those who retire and those who don't. The hazard ratio remains the same, and death rates are similar for those retiring at 60 and those retiring at 65.

Bottom line: As you plan your retirement, think about more than finances. Chapter 3 lays out in detail why delaying Social Security benefits until you are 66 or 70 is, without question, the more financially-literate decision. Further, mortality statistics indicate that delaying retirement has the higher benefit of likely keeping you alive longer.

But whether people intuitively know that working longer is good for them psychologically or financially, experts predict that people 55 and older will comprise 25 percent of the workforce by 2020, according to the Bureau of Labor Statistics.

Who Do You Want to Become?

Many people have the job they wanted and prepared for. They got all the utility they could wring out of their career choices and can't imagine having done anything else. Another group of persons fell into their jobs by accident and felt they had to keep those unfulfilling jobs to pay the rent. But even those with high job satisfaction have to acknowledge that, at some point, their firms no longer really want them, and unless they want to play golf or watch TV all day, a second career might be just the ticket. Besides, a new income stream can't hurt, and if you are self-employed, there is no age limit.

A growing problem is ageism — companies firing workers 55 and older without having a concrete reason, simply due to the perception that someone younger would do a better job, a sentiment that everyone knows is politically incorrect. Sometimes a worker, whether a hands-on laborer or office professional, gets sterling annual reviews for years on end, and suddenly one bad one — and dismissal. Many older workers often don't fight back, demonstrating that they themselves buy into the younger-is-better idea, but a good deal do resist. According to *The New York Times*, "Age discrimination claims are on the rise as members of the post-World War II baby boom enter their 60s. Last year, 22,857 people filed age-related complaints with the federal Equal Employment Opportunity Commission, compared with 16,548 in 2006." You can see the statistics on workplace discrimination charges on the basis of age (race, sex, color, religion, disability, retaliation, etc.) at the government website of the US Equal Opportunity Commission, EEOC.gov/eeoc/statistics/enforcement/charges.cfm. To file a case, call (800) 669-4000, (800) 669-6820 (TTY).

Working After Retirement

The AARP monthly magazine and many other publications trumpet second-time-around jobs for retirees, some of which enable you to work within your field of expertise, and others that take some preparation that you may be able to get an employer to sponsor.

Example 1: Upon a retirement, a bank clerk would like to work with dogs and gets her bank to make her a small business loan to pay for education and equipment — professional dog-bathing sink, grooming table, clippers, etc.

Example 2: A man retires from a major computer company. He has enough income for retirement, but chooses to donate his time to helping blind people use their computers. He keeps up with the technology and troubleshoots and upgrades their equipment using donated write-offs from his previous employer. He charges nothing, but his wife is grateful he is busy most days — his job gets him out of the house, giving him a sense of personal satisfaction.

Example 3: You have skill with numbers, but no real training. You take the H&R Block income tax course in how to help people prepare their tax returns. It's not a high-paying job — $8 to $12/hour — but it's seasonal, starting in late January and ending after tax season, a schedule that may suit you.

You can search for jobs that offer on-the-job training, but be careful — some are scams that charge you for training that is second-rate and then never deliver the job. Assuming you have little transferable skills, possible employment opportunities may include seeking work as a receptionist or with a temp firm, bartending at a golf and country club, or working in retail. If you have a higher education, you may qualify for becoming an online college degree-program instructor, or even pick up part-time work as a tutor. On-line degrees were pioneered by the University of Phoenix, but the industry has now expanded to hundreds of institutions. The classic *US News and World Report* ranking of the ten best colleges has now been joined by the ten best online educational institutions (published each January).

Instead of being an instructor, you could be a student. Or, with hands-on training at your own expense, you can train to be a sommelier (wine steward) in a fancy restaurant, a butler, or a real estate agent. If you are talented, you can buy a few books to learn how to set up shop as an organizer (closets and pantries) or as a home-for-sale stager.

Some companies prefer older workers, or are at least those who are elder-friendly. Not surprisingly, many of the best jobs for retirees are also the best jobs for people of any age — in the medical care industry. In the book *Great Jobs for Everyone 50+*, author Kerry Hannon divides jobs for seniors into ten categories that take into account existing skill-level and other factors. According to Hannon, the best-paying jobs for seniors include dietician/nutritionist and market-research surveyor.

Changing Jobs Before Retirement

The secret to finding a second career after your first career is to take an honest look at your interests and capabilities. Maybe you would like to write novels or paint oil paintings, but would anyone buy them? Chances are these are hobbies, not second careers. The heart-warming magazine articles fail to note that the vast majority of retirees need to work to get income, because their pension and Social Security is not sufficient to support the lifestyle they would like to have.

While taking that honest look at your interests and *capabilities,* run your eye down a list of occupations and don't be too hasty in rejecting anything. Wikipedia has lists organized by type (entertainment, medical, technology, etc.) and ChronicleCareer Library.com offers an alphabetical list of over 2000 occupations. The State of California has a list of 924 occupations that shows salaries and, in many cases, a video (CaCareerZone.org/ occupations/list).

The Bureau of Labor Statistics (BLS.gov/oes/current/oes_ stru.htm) lists occupations with a breakout of all the variations of the job description — how many persons employed in the field, and what they pay based on where you live. For example, choosing the category, "Hosts and Hostesses, Restaurant, Lounge, and Coffee Shop" produces the information that as of May 2012, 341,000 persons were in this occupation, mostly in restaurants, and they earned an average wage of $9.41/hour. Clicking on the job description, "Nonfarm Animal Caretakers" outside of vet offices — those who "Feed, water, groom, bathe, exercise, or otherwise care for pets and other nonfarm animals"— will reveal that 150,000 are employed in the field, making an average $10.75/hour. If you take a look at geographical distribution, you'll find that in Tennessee, for example, there are 2,350 persons employed in this category, and their average annual wage is $21,340. You can have quite a lot fun looking through these occupations with your friends and relatives.

Job coaches will tell you that you need to do some soul-searching before you are psychologically ready for a career change. Self-assessment tests are available online, but again, many require a name and e-mail address, and that opens you up to being pestered. Still, deleting some unwanted e-mails in order to find career-advisement that fits your particular needs is worth the time.

Step 1 is to be realistic, but to also think outside the box. It makes a lot more sense to imagine being a pastry chef if you are now a lawyer than becoming a lawyer if you are now a pastry chef, but you must be sure to use your imagination. You may like the job, but would you really be good at it? And again, conversely, you may be well-suited to the job, but do you think you'd like it? Picking a second career because of an impractical (or overly-practical) self-assessment will turn you into a job-hopper, not a second-careerist.

Step 2 is to not only make an inventory of the skills you have developed over your lifetime so far, but to value them properly. The worst phrases here are "I was only a housewife" and "I was only a factory worker." Housewifery implies organizational and logistical skills, and factory work may also imply logistical skills, mechanical skills, quality-control consciousness, and sensitivity to workplace safety.

Step 3 is to try it on for size. Visit the workplace and interview people who now have the job you think you want. You may love animals and want to work in a veterinary office, but are you prepared to see abused animals and to assist in euthanasia? You may love police work and want to become a 911 dispatcher, but do you wilt under pressure? If you want to start your own business, prepare a business plan and take it to an accountant or business planner for a brutally honest assessment. You may have to think again.

Step 4 is to look at the money-side of things. Many new jobs require additional education or training. Can you afford it, and can you afford to forego a paycheck for long enough to get the training you will need? If you are starting a business, do you have enough capital? Chances are you'll need more than you think. Be aware that running out of initial capital is the single biggest cause of new business failures.

The final step is to evaluate whether you can prepare a step-by-step plan to get from here to there. Once you've done your soul-searching, assessed your aptitude, and narrowed down your choice, you are ready to start the real work. Before embarking on any

TABLE 2-1: MOST JOBS AVAILABLE

Occupation	No. of New Jobs (Projected) 2012-2022	2012 Median Pay
Personal Care Aides	580,800	$19,910
Registered Nurses	526,800	$65,470
Retail Salespersons	434,700	$21,110
Home Health Aides	424,200	$20,820
Food Preparation/Service	421,900	$18,260
Nursing Assistants	312,200	$24,420
Secretary and Administrative Assistant	307,800	$32,410

TABLE 2-2: FASTEST GROWING OCCUPATIONS

Occupation	Projected Growth Rate 2012-2022	2012 Median Pay
Industrial-Organizational Psychologists	53%	$83,580
Personal Care	49%	$19,910
Home Health Aides	48%	$20,820
Insulation Workers, Mechanical	47%	$39,170
Interpreters and Translators	46%	$45,430
Diagnostic Medical Sonographers	46%	$65,860
Brick and Stone Mason helpers	43%	$28,220
Occupational Therapy Assistants	43%	$53,240

new education and training to get the credentials you will need, find out whether there are actually any jobs in the field. You may think you would be a splendid symphony orchestra conductor, but there are only about 1,200 symphony orchestras in the United States and the qualification-slope is steep. You also want to know how much the dream-job pays. Is there a commute involved, and if so, how will this affect your lifestyle? Will the hours interfere with your quality of life?

A good source is the Department of Labor's *Occupational Outlook Handbook*. The US Bureau of Labor statistics webiste, BLS. gov/ooh/ — the source of Tables 2-1, 2-2, and 2-3) — details the twenty most plentiful jobs in each field, the fastest twenty growing occupations, and the twenty highest paid. The most new jobs are for registered nurses, retail sales, home health aides, and personal care aides. Work in healthcare also makes the list of fastest growing occupation segment.

TABLE 2-3: HIGHEST PAID	
Occupation	**2012 Median Pay**
1. Oral and Maxillofacial Surgeons	=/>$187,200
8. Psychiatrists	$173,330
11. Chief Executives	$168,140
14. Nurse Anesthetists	$148,160
16. Petroleum Engineers	$130,280
18. Air Traffic Controllers	$122,530
19. Computer and Information Systems Managers	$120,950
20. Marketing Managers	$119,480

Fourteen of the top twenty, highest-paying jobs are medical/dental including surgeons, obstetricians and gynecologists, anesthesiologists, and family practitioners. While you can possibly get into medical school at 55, you would probably have to pay full tuition price. Are you good with computers? Most 15-year-olds are pretty good, too, but at a higher level, computer and system managers are 19th on the list and earn $120,950.

Starting Your Own Business after Retirement

If you can't bear the thought of cubicle life or ever working for another boss, take an inventory of your skills, including your organizational skills. After all, not everyone is educationally equipped to write a business plan that includes sales and marketing, public relations, finance, accounting, and product quality control, among other considerations associated with going into business for yourself.

Again, you are not alone. Numerous organizations will help you, including SCORE, which used to be named the Service Corps of Retired Executives. If you will be retiring with plenty of income, you may want to become a mentor to others seeking to start their own business (SCORE.org/mentors), or if you are the one seeking free advice on starting a business, you can speak directly with a SCORE expert at (800) 634-0245. They can help you with important start-up details, like getting funding from the Small Business Administration (SBA.gov, 800-827-5722). Another mentoring service organization is MicroMentor.org. Some organizations specialize in offering help to women entrepreneurs, including the Association of Women's Business Centers at AWBC.biz, (202)

552.8732; Women of Power — Black Enterprise at BlackEnterprise. com, (212) 242-8000; eWomenNetwork.com, (972) 620-9995; National Women Business Owners Corporation at NWBOC.org, (800) 675-5066; and National Association of Women Business Owners, NAWBO.org, (800) 556-2926.

Before starting your own business, you should decide how much complexity you can handle. Highly complex enterprises include franchising, which is fraught with legal contracts and requires you to conform to the franchisor's values and rules. Another complex business is direct sales. Think Avon Lady, although direct selling has moved online these days, and you could build a website selling kites or black walnuts, where you collect the orders and the manufacturer or producer makes the delivery (fulfillment).

Real estate is a good idea if you have some starting capital. Home prices fell 30 percent from 2006 to 2012 and began to recover only in 2013. Big companies went fishing for blocks of houses to buy as an investment, and you can, too. Depending on your region, there is an inventory of cheap properties available for renovation and rental or re-sale. You have to be able to juggle several things at once — financial paperwork, contractors and sub-contractors, decorators, real estate agents, and tenants if you decide to rent instead of sell. Flipping houses can be dirty, labor intensive, and expensive, and you have to be up to it. Maybe becoming a home property appraiser or inspector would be less stressful, although you have to take a course and obtain a license.

At the more simple level, you can take a course in woodworking and produce hand-made furniture in your workshop, or a course in quilting and sell quilts at fairs or online. Pet-sitting is a newly emerging occupation, either in your own home or at the pet-owner's home, and it doesn't take any training — just an affinity for animals.

If you live in a big city, you can curb-trawl for good stuff that people throw away to sell to antique dealers and second-hand shops. You can scan books with a smart phone at church sales and fairs to get the ISBN number and quickly see if the book you are holding at 50¢ might actually fetch $50 on Amazon.com. In addition to Christine Miller's groundbreaking, *How to Sell Books on Amazon*, ironically, you can now find books on how to find books on eBay and sell them on Amazon.

Now we have mentioned the magic word: eBay. Selling on eBay has become a cottage industry in the United States, and you don't have to pay to take a course — eBay offers you free, online tutorials. A big drawback if you are finding or making you own products and doing your own shipping is that shipping costs are very high these days, so it pays to buy a scale and learn the actual shipping cost before you advertise "free shipping," which eBay recommends because buyers like it so much.

There's nothing like the sense of liberty you get when you are your own boss at last. And that's exactly the problem: You value that liberty so much that you are willing to overlook serious business failures in order to keep it.

Which brings us to the leading cause of new, small business failure: running out of start-up capital before your product or service is self-supporting. You may be in a state of denial that the demand for your product is high enough to let you enter the industry, or that you have a firm grip on your supply costs and supplier reliability. Often it happens that sales are more or less equal to costs, so your living expenses (and taxes) are coming out of savings. This is one thing when you are 22 and living in your parents' basement, but an entirely different situation when you are 60 and have your own kids living in the basement. The numbers have to be realistic and work upfront before you start, including a big fudge-factor for "estimation error." And beware of quitting your job to provide a product or service to your employer. The American landscape is littered with workers who made a big initial gain as a sub-contractor to their employer, but when that employer moved on, they had no other customers.

The second biggest cause of new business failure is being a bad manager. You can get the spreadsheet numbers right, but have personality traits that sabotage your business. On one side are the people-pleasers who underprice their products and services in order to seek approval from everyone — even bad suppliers, rude customers, and lazy employees. On the other side are the self-righteous, I'm-the-boss types who are perfectionists and can't get out of everyone else's way and let them get on with their jobs. Still another type is the person so convinced that the product is sure to be a top-seller, that he/she turns a blind eye to the financial realities. But it's not the job of the bookkeeper or the accountant to evaluate financial performance. Venture capitalists almost always want to install a new CEO in the enterprises in which they invest specifically because the entrepreneur is hardly ever a good manager or bookkeeper, especially if he/she is an inventor.

The third cause of new business failure is lack of adaptability. You had a five-year strategic plan but the market changed entirely in year three. Let's say you opened a bookstore in a small town and then along came the Kindle, or you opened a hardware store and Home Depot opened up ten miles away. Not only do you have to cope with the business cycle and changing customer tastes, you have to wrestle with new technology, which offers an especially powerful form of competition.

The final reason new businesses fail is, surprisingly, success. Good initial results make the business-owner over-expand operations to new products or new markets, usually borrowing too much to do so. Sometimes the borrowing is from family and friends who see existing success but are unqualified to judge whether that success can realistically be leveraged into a bigger enterprise.

Employment Resources

Online job banks for retired and semi-retired boomers abound. To help you get started, here are some of the more popular and comprehensive sites:

RetirementJobs.com, which charges a small membership fee, is one of the biggest sites for retirees who want to keep working in the same industry or change environment altogether.

SeniorJobBank.org, (866) 562-2627, has been recommended in such publications as *Forbes*, *The Saturday Evening Post*, and *BusinessWeek*, as well as on CNN.com and About.com.

Encore.org, (415) 430-0141, is an organization established in 1998 that aims to help people find a self-fulfilling, second career. It offers job listings, education and training resources, and a get-started guide. You can also try to answer the "big questions" about your purpose in life and how to find it at the Encore affiliated site, BigQuestionsOnline.com/questions.

Workforce50.com "arms the older workforce with employment resources and career information to achieve their goals."

USAjobs.gov offers government, full-time and contract employment for retired federal and non-federal employees, veterans, individuals with disabilities, and senior executives.

For the retiring, high-level, executive boomer, their wealth of experience is much sought after in the realms of consulting and contract work. The following sites offer advisement and act as intermediaries, finding employment opportunities commensurate with your field and level of expertise.

Execunet.com, (800) 637-3126, is a private membership community offering new opportunities to the executive-level job seeker.

NewDirections.com, (617) 523-7775, a Boston-based firm, is geared toward helping high-level executives re-invent themselves, both in late career and in retirement.

BoomersConsultingLLC.com, (678) 476-8243, offers mid- to senior-level, full-time and consulting opportunities within the engineering, healthcare, and information technology industries.

YourEncore.com, (609) 534-5388, offers top-notch employment opportunities ranging from one-time consulting assignments to projects lasting a year or more.

Don't think about the "right" time to retire until you've decided how you'll spend your time afterward — and how you'll finance that time. Be sure to keep the following retirement-planning "do's and don'ts" in mind:

DaVINCI DO'S

- Think twice about early retirement. Not only does it significantly reduce your Social Security benefit, but studies show that it negatively affects lifespan. Staying active in the workforce not only earns you money today and an increased benefit in the future, but helps sustain mental acuity, physical health, combats depression, and makes for an overall happier and more well-balanced lifestyle.

- If you do find that you need to change jobs before retirement, take an honest-to-goodness look at your interests and abilities, being sure to choose a job that reconciles the two. On-line assessment tests can be very helpful in narrowing down your options.

- If you are a high-level executive retiree, put your years of expertise to work as a consultant. You'd be surprised how many firms are looking for individuals just like you, with decades of invaluable experience to offer. The consulting firms are a great starting point.

DaVINCI DON'TS

- Better late than never. Even if you're nearing retirement, don't think that it's too late to start planning. There are numerous resources throughout this book to help you chart your course at any stage.

- If you're plan is to start a new business late in your working career, don't make any firm decisions until you've decided exactly how much complexity you can handle. Many businesses fail within the first year, and losing a chunk of your nest egg is much easier to swallow at 23 than it is at 53.

- Don't consider retirement planning a strictly financial endeavor. Think about the many ways you'll be spending your time — days can be long without purposeful and meaningful activities that are necessary to achieve balance in your life, while maintaining both your physical and mental vitality.

Social Security

3

AT THE TIME SOCIAL Security was passed into law in 1935, half of all retirees lived below the poverty level. The primary goal of Social Security was to alleviate that poverty, and later to offer benefits to the disabled. Social Security was never intended to be a retirement program, but rather a supplement to the pensions and savings of individuals.

A great many conceptual errors surround Social Security, even today. First of all, it's an insurance trust that is funded by annual payroll taxes of both workers and employers — not a Ponzi scheme, as some charge. In fact, the actual fund is named the Old-Age and Survivors Insurance Trust Fund. Former Social Security Administrator Jason Fichtner says, "It was never intended to be the sole means for people to live off of in retirement. It's insurance against the possibility that you'll run out of saving by living too long." The personal-responsibility aspect of the program is that individuals are assumed to have some personal savings. "Gimmicks that treat

Social Security as a lottery where big bucks can be won not only negatively affect the solvency of the program but also undermine the societal support for Social Security."

Critics who charge that Social Security is a Ponzi scheme are not applying the concept correctly. A Ponzi scheme operator claims the rate of return on an investment is extraordinarily high because of his special skills, but in actuality, he simply repays old investors with fresh money from new investors. Bernie Madoff operated a Ponzi scheme. Such schemes fail when the supply of new investors dries up, or a government regulatory agency finds fraud in an audit. Fraud and the intent to defraud are integral to Ponzi schemes. Fraud takes the form of promising, for instance, a 20 percent return when no-risk or low-risk returns are far lower; fraud is detected by the auditor looking into the exact investments in the portfolio to determine the actual rate of return — something the SEC failed to do in the Madoff case.

It is true that, parallel to the Ponzi methodology in one respect, Social Security pays out benefits to current recipients almost entirely from funds collected from new participants, while the trust fund continues to grow. But there is no fraud or intent to defraud; the Social Security Administration (SSA) doesn't promise extraordinary return rates — the return on participants' funds is the same for everyone, and the books are completely transparent. The Office of the Inspector General audits Social Security every year, and the audits can be seen by everyone online. In fact, audits are directed not only to the management of the fund, but also to fraud, waste, and abuse by recipients.

The insurance aspect of Social Security is straightforward. With typical, commercial insurance, you pay a premium along with many others and the insurance company pools those funds on the expectation, backed up by massive amounts of statistics, that only a fraction of the pooled funds will be appropriated toward claims. Insurance transfers the risk of any single bad event over a larger pool of those at the same risk of anything from car accidents to home fires, shipwrecks, and so on. Insurance companies scale the amount of premium you pay to the amount of the claim you could ultimately make, but the amount of premium you pay will likely be far less than your claim if you are unlucky enough to need an insurance payout. If you insure your car in January and it's totaled in February, you will have only made a single premium payment, but you will collect the full face value of the policy (less the deductible).

As stated, the insurance company gets the rest of the money beyond what you paid in from the pooled funds, including those who insured at the same time as you, those who began afterward, and those who started paying in ten years ago. Additional capital is generated by the return on the invested funds. Again, this system functions exactly the same as Social Security. The only difference is that commercial insurance policies are closed-ended — the maximum amount you can get by reporting a claim is fixed, whether it's your car, your house, or your life.

But Social Security is open-ended — you will receive benefits until you die. It would have been heartless and politically unacceptable to say a person could receive benefits from 62 to, say, 85, and then benefits would end. In fact, the very first person to receive Social Security benefits was Ida Mae Miller, who had paid $24.75 in Social Security contributions by the time of her retirement in 1939, but received $22,888.92 in benefits by the time she died at 100 in 1975.

As long as the population of wage-earners continues to rise and to make contributions to the trust fund, Social Security will be funded. Social Security cannot borrow money in its own name, so its only funding sources are the current payroll taxes and the trust fund. Many people do not understand this point — Social Security does not contribute to the federal budget deficit. Legally, it cannot, since it cannot borrow.

The Social Security Trust Fund had $2.8 trillion by the end of June 2014, but demographic changes — the rise in the baby boomer retirement population — means that future taxes are projected to fall short of the collective payments in coming years. By 2033, benefits would have to be reduced by 23 percent if the tax rate is not raised. According to Steve Goss, chief actuary for the SSA, taxes paid into the system will be 4.7 percent of GDP by 2030, but payments will be 6.1 percent. Closing the gap requires raising the payroll tax or cutting benefits — but cutting benefits is not the same thing as "Social Security going broke" or ending benefits altogether, as fear-mongers claim. As of year-end 2013, the FICA (Federal Insurance Contributions Act, or payroll tax) rate was 6.2 percent and the Medicare tax rate was 1.45 percent.

It's of more than passing interest that reforming immigration and raising employment generally would capture more Social Security taxes and delay tapping the trust fund. Economists estimate that the "gray-market economy" — people working off the books — is about $10 billion. The FICA tax on $10 billion would be $620 million, and that's not chickenfeed.

The Real Social Security Problem

The true Social Security dilemma is not Social Security itself — it's Medicare/Medicaid. The $23 trillion in unfunded Social Security liabilities that will appear by 2033 is today about 1.4 percent of the GDP, or four percent of total taxable payrolls. By 2033, the US GDP will be a higher number, if history is a guide.

Scare-stories about Social Security running out of money always include the unfunded liabilities of Medicare/Medicaid and the Medicare Prescription Drug Program as well. Combining the three programs misrepresents the issues. And the combined liability is quoted anywhere from $120 trillion up to $178 trillion, depending upon the assumptions of the writer. But as noted, Social Security itself is not in dire straits, and, in fact, will almost certainly go into the black when the baby-boom generation leaves the scene. Of the total unfunded liability out into the distant future, the unfunded Social Security component is about $23.1 trillion, falling to $9.6 trillion by 2087. If you like actuarial analysis, you can see the numbers (and projection assumptions) for yourself in the 2013 annual report of the board of trustees of the Federal Old-Age and Survivors Insurance and Federal Disability Insurance Trust Fund (SSA.gov/oact/tr/2013/tr2013.pdf).

Calculating unfunded liabilities is a tricky business that relies on assumptions about demographic changes, such as birth rates, immigration, and longevity, among other things, and is still a work-in-progress. It's true that in 2013, the Social Security trustees raised the amount of the unfunded liability over the next 75 years by $1 trillion to $9.6 trillion. Unfunded liabilities are a serious matter — they represent benefits promised to people that will not be funded by the tax revenues currently in place.

However, it's important not to tar Social Security with Medicare's brush. The probability of Social Security being eliminated altogether is, for all practical purposes: zero. Politicians call it the "third rail" of politics, meaning it's too electrically-charged to touch or tamper with.

In fact, it's conceptually wrong to regard Social Security in the context of any other public welfare issue, such as immigration. It is not true that illegal immigrants can collect Social Security benefits; federal law prohibits paying Social Security benefits to illegal immigrants. Social Security stands alone — it is self-supporting and independent. If you hear a story about Social Security that seems fishy, you can check it out at SSA.gov, Snopes.com, or UrbanLegends.com.

Final Debunking

It's a myth that when Social Security was founded, the retirement age of 65 was selected because so few would be around to collect it. This is simply not true and reflects a distrust of government that is unwarranted in this case.

When the Social Security Act (originally the Economic Security Act) was signed in August 1935, the statisticians projected that that 54 percent of men born in 1940 would, in fact, live to 65 if they made it past 21. They would then have another 12.7 years, for a total life expectancy of 77.7 years. For women, 61 percent would live to 65 if they made it past 21, and they would have an additional 14.7 years (living to 79.7 years). It is therefore not historically accurate that the original Social Security retirement age of 65 was

TABLE 3-1: LIFE EXPECTANCY FOR SOCIAL SECURITY

Year Cohort Turned 65	Percentage of Population Surviving from Age 21 to Age 65		Average Remaining Life Expectancy for Those Surviving to Age 65	
	Male	Female	Male	Female
1940	53.9	60.6	12.7	14.7
1950	56.2	65.5	13.1	16.2
1960	60.1	71.3	13.2	17.4
1970	63.7	76.9	13.8	18.6
1980	67.8	80.9	14.6	19.1
1990	72.3	83.6	15.3	19.6

Source: http://www.ssa.gov/history/lifeexpect.html

selected because hardly anyone would be left to collect. For the most part, the SSA did have a grip on the data.

What they may not have known was that the survival rate of those who made it to 21 would rise from 54 percent to 72.3 percent for men, and from 60.6 percent to 83.6 percent for women over the next 50 years.

How it Works in Practice

When you are 59, and thus nearing the conventional retirement age, the SSA will start sending you an annual statement that arrives around your birthday and spells out the amount you will receive if you retire at each of several possible ages. You don't have to wait until you're 59 to see the amounts — you can check it out at the SSA website, SSA.gov/estimator. You get a lesser amount if you retire at age 62 than if you wait until you are 66 (or 67 if you were born after 1954), and you get the biggest amount if you wait until you are 70. These benchmark ages were valid as of the 2013 year-end and may change.

The Social Security Administration uses an index to calculate your benefits. The indexing has the effect of lifting up your benefit if you were lower-paid, and limiting it if you were highly paid. Lower and higher are judged in comparison to the national average. In other words, indexing brings your actual earnings closer to the current wage level in each of the 35 years covered. This is a bit complicated, but if you think about it, it's a leveling process that is fairer to everyone — high earners get their earnings adjusted downward and still get higher Social Security benefits, but not disproportionately. Lower earners get a higher benefit by adjusting their earnings closer to the national average. In addition, and equally important, the indexing adjusts earlier years for subsequent wage inflation.

The SSA publishes wage inflation factors every year. The number you care about is the one published the year you turn 60, because your index number remains the same, at one, for every year after that. In other words, you don't get any credit for wage inflation after age 60, although your benefits, once you start collecting them, are adjusted for cost-of-living increases.

The average benefit was $1,230 as of 2013, but averages can disguise a wide range of other pertinent data. The maximum in 2013 for someone retiring at age 62 was $1,923, but at the full retirement age of 66, it was $2,533. If you retired at age 70 in 2013, the maximum benefit was $3,350.

How Your Social Security Benefit is Calculated

In order to calculate an applicant's benefit, an *indexing factor* is created that brings past-years' wages to the current equivalent for

TABLE 3-2: NATIONAL AVERAGE WAGE INDEXING SERIES, 1951-2012

Year	National Avg. Wage Index	Year	National Avg. Wage Index	Year	National Avg. Wage Index
1951	2,799.16	1976	9,226.48	2001	32,921.92
1952	2,973.32	1977	9,779.44	2002	33,252.09
1953	3,139.44	1978	10,556.03	2003	34,064.95
1954	3,155.64	1979	11,479.46	2004	35,648.55
1955	3,301.44	1980	12,513.46	2005	36,952.94
1956	3,532.36	1981	13,773.10	2006	38,651.41
1957	3,641.72	1982	14,531.34	2007	40,405.48
1958	3,673.80	1983	15,239.24	2008	41,334.97
1959	3,855.80	1984	16,135.07	2009	40,711.61
1960	4,007.12	1985	16,822.51	2010	41,673.83
1961	4,086.76	1986	17,321.82	2011	42,979.61
1962	4,291.40	1987	18,426.51	2012	44,321.67
1963	4,396.64	1988	19,334.04		
1964	4,576.32	1989	20,099.55		
1965	4,658.72	1990	21,027.98		
1966	4,938.36	1991	21,811.60		
1967	5,213.44	1992	22,935.42		
1968	5,571.76	1993	23,132.67		
1969	5,893.76	1994	23,753.53		
1970	6,186.24	1995	24,705.66		
1971	6,497.08	1996	25,913.90		
1972	7,133.80	1997	27,426.00		
1973	7,580.16	1998	28,861.44		
1974	8,030.76	1999	30,469.84		
1975	8,630.92	2000	32,154.82		

Source: http://www.ssa.gov/oact/COLA/AWI.html

those years up until the applicant turns 60. This is the factor referred to in Table 3-3.

This indexing factor is calculated by taking the national average wage index for the year in which the applicant turns 60 and dividing it by the national average wage index for each previous year, starting from when the individual began working. Given that eligibility for Social Security benefits is age 62, and we are currently in 2014, the national average wage index of $44,321.67 for 2012 is used — that of the year the applicant turns 60.

The following table from the SSA website lists the national-average-wage indices from 1951–2012:

Taking a look at **Case A** in Table 3-3 from the SSA webpage (SSA.gov/oact/progdata/retirebenefit1.html), the start year is 1974 and the retirement year is 2014. Based on the indexing series, the average wage for 2012 ($44,321.67) divided by the average wage for 1974 ($8,030.76), yields an indexing factor of 5.5190. That calculation is done for each the 35 years covered, resulting in a cumulative total and an average over all those months (35 years times 12 months per year = 420 months) in order to obtain an **Average Indexed Monthly Earnings** (AIME).

This is the main calculation, but there's more. After finding your AIME, the SSA applies the **Age-At-Retirement Modification.** This is a three-step process that converts your AIME into benefits by using two **bend points**. This sounds strange, but stay with it, because bend points could be your best friend — they are the adjustments that give the lower-paid a bigger slice of replacement income than higher-income workers get. This is the "progressive" part of the arrangement. For instance, if everyone got 40 percent of their average monthly income, the higher-paid would get an absolute dollar amount many times greater than what lower-paid workers would get. The bend points skew the final benefit to be paid, which is known as the **Primary Insurance Amount** (PIA), and is in favor of lower-wage workers.

There are two bend points, and the ones you care about are the ones published for the year you turn 62, when it becomes a fixed number for you. Bend points are adjusted for inflation each year (although that may change). The bend points published by the Social Security Administration for those turning 62 in 2014 are $816 and $4,917.

TABLE 3-3: EARNINGS BEFORE AND AFTER INDEXING

Year	Case A, born in 1952		
	Nominal Earnings	Indexing Factor	Indexed Earnings
1974	$7,509	5.5190	$41,442
1975	8,095	5.1352	41,570
1976	8,681	4.8037	41,701
1977	9,230	4.5321	41,832
1978	9,994	4.1987	41,962
1979	10,903	3.8610	42,096
1980	11,921	3.5419	42,223
1981	13,162	3.2180	42,355
1982	13,930	3.0501	42,488
1983	14,653	2.9084	42,617
1984	15,562	2.7469	42,748
1985	16,275	2.6347	42,879
1986	16,809	2.5587	43,010
1987	17,935	2.4053	43,139
1988	18,875	2.2924	43,269
1989	19,682	2.2051	43,401
1990	20,653	2.1077	43,531
1991	21,487	2.0320	43,662
1992	22,662	1.9325	43,793
1993	22,925	1.9160	43,924
1994	23,610	1.8659	44,054
1995	24,630	1.7940	44,186
1996	25,911	1.7103	44,317
1997	27,503	1.6160	44,446
1998	29,028	1.5357	44,577
1999	30,735	1.4546	44,707
2000	32,530	1.3784	44,839
2001	33,403	1.3463	44,969
2002	33,836	1.3329	45,100
2003	34,764	1.3011	45,231
2004	36,485	1.2433	45,362
2005	37,929	1.1994	45,492
2006	39,786	1.1467	45,623
2007	41,711	1.0969	45,754
2008	42,792	1.0723	45,884
2009	42,267	1.0887	46,015
2010	43,389	1.0635	46,146
2011	44,875	1.0312	46,276
2012	46,407	1.0000	46,407
2013	47,068	1.0000	47,068
		Highest-35 total	1,551,588
		AIME	3,694

So, for the individual who turns 62 in 2014, his or her PIA will be the sum of:

(a) 90 percent of the first $816 of average indexed monthly earnings, plus

(b) 32 percent of average indexed monthly earnings over $816 up to $4,917, plus

(c) 15 percent of average indexed monthly earnings over $4,917.

The Social Security Administration webpage, SocialSecurity.gov/OACT/COLA/piaformula.html, defines and explains PIA and bend point calculations.

The Best Age to Apply

Everyone knows you get a bigger monthly check the longer you wait to apply. But there are really two questions you need to answer in figuring out the best age to apply: (1) How much money will I get? and (2) How long will I live?

The money amount you get by taking early Social Security at age 62 is about 25 percent lower than if you wait until you are 66. If you wait until you are 70, you get about eight percent more for every year you wait. Government notes and bonds all yield less than eight percent — you'd have to be an investment wizard to do better. Besides, your spouse will get a higher survivor's benefit if you wait until 66 and even more if you wait until 70.

But if you are in bad health or your family history suggests you won't make it much past your early 70s, you could be trying to save up that eight percent per annum for only a few short years.

Let's say your benefit at age 62 is equal to $1,200 (near the national average). If you accept your benefits then, that's the amount you will get for the remainder of your life, plus whatever inflation adjustment, even if you live to 100. If you wait until you are 66, your monthly benefit is $1,600, and again, that amount never goes up except through inflation adjustment. But if you wait to apply for benefits until you are 70, you will get a whopping $2,110, or 76 percent more than at age 62. This is not a sum of money to sneeze at.

TABLE 3-4: MONTHLY BENEFITS				
Age 62	**Age 63–65**	**Age 66**	**Age 66–70**	**Age 70**
$1,200	$1,200	$1,600	$1,600	$2,110

TABLE 3-5: MONTHLY BENEFITS			
	Age 62	**Age 66**	**Age 70**
Monthly	$1,200	$1,600	$2,110
Cumulative at Age 78	$230,400	$230,400	$202,560
Cumulative At Age 90	$403,200	$460,800	$506,400

Monthly Benefits at Retirement Age

The first thing to notice about this table is that it doesn't do you any good to wait to age 63 — you will still get the same amount as you would at 62. The same thing holds for ages 66–70. At age 69, you still get the age 66 benefit.

Now consider the cumulative totals. If you take the age 62 version for $1,200 and live to 78 (16 years), you will have received $230,400 overall. If you take the age 66 version for $1,600 and live to 78 (12 years), you will have received the same amount, $230,400. If you wait until you are 70 to start getting benefits of $2,110 and live to 78, your total amount is $202,560. But if you were to live to 90 (an additional 20 years), your total would be $506,400.

Cumulative Benefits by Retirement Start Age

Therefore, it really does matter how long you will live. As addressed in Chapter 1, you can get an estimate of your life expectancy on numerous websites. Here are two more: LivingTo100.com and Apps.BlueZones.com/vitality.

Because longevity is rising, every advisor will tell you the best policy is to wait until you are 70 to apply for Social Security. But despite this advice, the AARP reports that only 14.3 percent of men and 9.7 percent of women wait until age 66, and even fewer wait until 70 — only between one and three percent.

The Breakeven

Filing at 62 gets you money in the bank faster, but at the expense of a lower monthly payment for the rest of your life. Waiting until you are 70 gives you a higher monthly payment, but less money cumulatively due to a shorter remaining lifespan.

According to AARP, if you wait until your "full retirement age," or FRA (66 for people born from 1943 through 1954; 67 thereafter), your benefit is one-third larger than if you take it at 62. If you wait until you are 70, your benefit will be 76 percent larger than if taken at 62. Notice that these numbers don't agree with some of the other numbers about benefits in this chapter. That's because different calculations make different assumptions about where your benefit falls on the sliding Social Security scale. Some estimates make the 62–66 delay worth 25 percent more, and others, like AARP, make it one-third more. The 66–70 delay can be 60 percent or 85 percent, depending on what you've earned over the 35-year calculation period. Don't let these discrepancies bother you. They do not imply there is anything tricky going on. The important thing is to go to the Social Security site (SSA.gov/planners) and figure out the gains percentage for your own circumstances.

The longer you live, the more your own specific chart of benefits will matter — and chances are, you'll live a long time. The average 65-year-old can expect roughly 20 more years of life. Among that same group, 41 percent of women and 28 percent of men will live to age 90, and half of those women will make it to 95, as will one-third of the men.

According to Andy Landis in *Social Security: The Inside Story*, filing at 62 instead of 66 puts you "money ahead" until you are 78. At age 78, the person who waited until he was 66 has caught up and then goes on to get a higher monthly payment for the rest of his life. "The bottom line is that if you just want the most dollars from SSA and expect to live past age 78, file at 66, not 62."

- You should file at 62 if you expect to live to 70.

- You should file at 66 if you expect to live to 80.

- You should file at 70 if you expect to live to 90.

Spousal Benefit

Deciding at what age to apply for Social Security should include a consideration of spousal benefit. A spouse is a wife or husband, and includes divorced wives and husbands if the marriage lasted at least ten years. As a rule, Social Security accepts the definition of marriage that each state determines, including in some cases, common-law marriages. If the worker is already on Social Security, the spouse in entitled to:

- 35 percent of the benefit amount at age 62

- 50 percent of the benefit at age 66 (FRA)

- 50 percent of the benefit if caring for a child entitled to benefits

Divorced spouses can claim essentially the same benefits as current spouses if the marriage lasted at least ten years and the divorced claimant is currently unmarried. In the case of divorced spouses, the worker need not have claimed benefits for the divorced spouse to be able to claim benefits (such as sidestepping, resentful spouses who never retire in order to deprive the divorced spouse of benefits).

If You Are Single

Social Security benefits are gender neutral, even though a woman's life expectancy is longer than a man's. A man and a woman with identical earnings histories get exactly the same benefits. It is, therefore, clear that it's more beneficial for women to delay applying for Social Security, since they will be relying on it a lot longer. Here is a useful comparison from a CBS News press report:

"... a 62-year-old female has an average life expectancy of 84. If her full retirement benefit is $1,000:

TABLE 3-6: MONTHLY BENEFITS

	Female Files at 62	Female Files at 70	Benefit to Delaying
Avg. Life Expectancy Minus Five Years (Age 79)	$113,352	$105,618	−6.8%
Avg. Life Expectancy (Age 84)	$134,305	$150,421	12.0%
Avg. Life Expectancy Plus Five Years (Age 89)	$150,911	$186,906	23.9%
	Male Files at 62	**Male Files at 70**	**Benefit to Delaying**
Avg. Life Expectancy Minus Five Years (Age 76)	$98,423	$74,239	−24.6%
Avg. Life Expectancy (Age 81)	$122,295	$124,612	1.9%
Avg. Life Expectancy Plus Five Years (Age 86)	$141,434	$165,950	17.3%

Source: CBS Money Watch, http://www.cbsnews.com/news/how-single-filers-can-get-the-most-from-social-security/

- She will receive $750 per month if she files at age 62.

- She will receive $1,320 per month if she files at age 70.

A man of the same age gets the same benefits (assuming his full retirement benefit is also $1,000 per month). However, his average life expectancy is three years shorter. Table 3-6 shows how a three-year difference in life expectancies between women and men changes the overall strategy for filing."

Again, it's important to emphasize that the longer you think you will live — perhaps your parents and other close relatives have lived past 90 — you are still better off delaying your benefit until age 70. "In effect, delaying benefits is like buying longevity insurance. If you live longer than expected, you decrease the risk of running out of money. If you don't live longer than expected, you didn't need the money anyway."

Only 2–3 percent of those eligible for Social Security wait until they are 70. We are lacking noteworthy data that reflects why such a large proportion of people take the 25 percent haircut on their benefits by making their Social Security claim at age 62 instead of waiting. It's easier to understand for singles than for married couples — when you are single, you don't need to consider getting as much money as possible for your survivor.

SOME COOL LIFE-EXPECTANCY DATA

People over 65 are the fastest growing segment of the population. (Sociologists refer to a large population like this as a "cohort.") According to the US Census Bureau report, *The Older Population: 2010*, those 65 and older number 40.3 million — up 15.1 percent from the 2000 census. The total population is growing at a rate of 9.7 percent. The over-65 cohort is about 13 percent of the total population — not as much as the 25–44 years group (26.6 percent); however, that latter group is actually shrinking. The fastest growth is among those 85–94, up 29.9 percent, from 3.9 million in the 2000 census to 5.1 million in the 2010 census. Those who are 100 and older also increased — by 5.8 percent to 53,364 persons.

It seems crazy to forego 25 percent more income by filing early at age 62, but there is one way in which it is the financially-wise choice: if you are unemployed and permanently discouraged about the prospect of getting another job, and if you would have to withdraw money from a tax-deferred account like a traditional IRA. The tax rate on an IRA withdrawal is your standard income tax rate; the IRA only defers taxes, it doesn't eliminate them. You have to do the calculation, but federal and state income taxes on Social Security payments are almost certainly lower than the income taxes on your IRA savings. Roth plans are funded with after-tax dollars and should be kept until the last possible moment, since they continue racking up returns. Withdrawing $20,000 from an IRA costs you $5,000 in taxes if you are in the 25 percent tax bracket, while withdrawing from a Roth has no tax cost, but if you have both, keep the Roth for its earning power.

Four other reasons for making the early claim:

1. You have enough money to retire and the extra Social Security payment offers the opportunity for a few luxuries.

2. You do not have enough savings to retire and you need the money to get by.

3. You are afraid politicians will interfere with the payment schedules, but you hope to get grandfathered into the plan (meaning they may change the benefit schedule for upcoming generations but those already in the plan get to keep the benefits they have already claimed).

4. You don't need the Social Security benefit to live on, but you believe you have trading and investment skills and you can get a higher return in the stock or commodities markets than you "earn" by delaying your application for benefits. This may or may not be true. One good clue is to check your average annual return in trading/investing over the past ten years and the volatility of those returns. Is it better than eight percent per year and did it vary by no more than five percent?

To these reasons, we want to add a fifth: the sense of security and well-being that you get from receiving Social Security payments. The utility of having the Social Security payment, safe from prying political hands, is a quality-of-life matter.

Will you have enough money? The short answer for most people is no. Some people who earned exceptionally high incomes and others who were exceptionally frugal can say yes, but the majority of baby boomers failed to save enough for retirement, let alone extreme old age requiring specialized care. Assuming you live to the average 78.8 years, we should probably also assume that you will not still be earning income from a job. Some oldsters are still working, such as artists — Robert Redford was born in 1936 and Tony Bennett in 1926 — but it's not realistic to expect to work to the very end of your life.

Therefore, unless you are in desperate financial straits, wait until 66 to apply for Social Security benefits, and preferably until you are 70. It may seem too silly to mention, but unless you are really rich and decide not to accept Social Security at all, there is absolutely no reason to delay after age 70.

Cost-of-Living Adjustments (COLA)

Social Security beneficiaries complain that the cost-of-living adjustments, started in 1973, are not geared to realistic price inflation faced by ordinary people. In 2010 and 2011, there was no increase in benefits, on the grounds that inflation was zero. In 2014, the cost-of-living increase is 1.5 percent, or about $19, raising the average monthly benefit to $1,294.

- 2010   zero
- 2011   zero
- 2012   3.6%
- 2013   1.7%
- 2014   1.5%

This skimpy raise — less than the rise in the average cost of prescription drugs — generates anger. But the Social Security Act mandates the calculation methodology. First comes the Consumer Price Index for Urban Wage Earners and Clerical Workers, denoted as CPI-W and calculated monthly by the Bureau of Labor Statistics. The COLA for December of 2013 was calculated by taking the year-over-year percentage change in CPI-W from the third quarter (three months) over the third quarter of the year before. The exact calculation for the 2013 COLA is: (230.327 − 226.936) / 226.936 x 100 = 1.5 percent.

The skimpy COLA adjustment is not Social Security's fault — it's the fault of the CPI-W failing to represent the costs of real, live Social Security beneficiaries. It's a perfect case of one size does not fit all. The Bureau of Labor Statistics takes data comprised of about 200 items divided into eight categories (food, housing, apparel, transportation, medical care, recreation, education, and "other") and comes up with average price increases in each

TABLE 3-7: CPI-W FOR 2012-2013	2012	2013
July	225.568	230.084
August	227.056	230.359
September	228.184	230.537
Third quarter total	680.808	690.980
Average (rounded to the nearest 0.001)	226.936	230.327

Source: Social Security Administration, http://www.ssa.gov/oact/STATS/cpiw.html

category, smoothing away big differences in regional prices and other factors. The BLS admits the CPI is not a cost-of-living index.

The problem for Social Security beneficiaries is that they spend a great deal less on things like apparel and education than the hypothetical, average consumer, and a great deal more on medical costs. Retired and disabled people pay twice as much for healthcare as the average consumer, and transportation forms a higher percentage of their budgets, too. The justification for creating a special CPI for retired Social Security beneficiaries is obvious — and indeed the BLS does calculate a CPI-E for the elderly — but instead of a political move to replace the CPI-W with the CPI-E (described in Chapter 1), we are getting political proposals to introduce "chaining," the biggest controversy today.

What is chaining? It's a calculation methodology that makes perfect sense academically but has the side-effect of underestimating true consumer preferences. The core concept is that applying a fixed weight to each item in the shopping basket fails to account for changes in the quality of the items, and also the simple fact that rising prices drive consumers toward less costly substitutes. To keep counting items at fixed weight would therefore understate inflation. The classic case is pork vs. beef. If the price of pork goes up, consumers substitute lower-cost beef. Under the fixed weight method, CPI inflation went up because the price of pork went up. Under the chained-CPI method, sufficient substitution of beef for pork would cause prices to appear lower, and subsequently, COLA to be lower, too. At some point you are measuring the cost of survival, not the cost of living.

Critics of using chaining to determine Social Security COLA assert that the savings are trivial in the grand scheme of the US budget deficit, but truly meaningful to beneficiaries. The $25 or $45 difference in the monthly benefit can make the difference between taking all your medicines and doling them out in dosages less than prescribed. To claim that Social Security should be cut to reduce the US budget deficit is a fallacy, since Social Security is self-funded and outside the deficit process in the first place.

Social Security Optimization Strategies

Social Security seems relatively straightforward, but can quickly become impenetrably complex when the applicant has special circumstances. Former Social Security administrator Andy Landis writes that in his twelve years at the SSA, he saw some bizarre situations arising from super-complicated family structures — multiple marriages, several sets of children, and several equally plausible and legal Social Security payment outcomes. If you have a complicated family structure, especially if disabilities are involved, get ready to spend some time with an SSA-appointed advocate or a lawyer specializing in Social Security.

But some of the strategies for optimizing benefits are straightforward. If you Google "Social Security tricks," you will get over 34 million hits. Evidently that's a catchy title. But the number of real-life strategies is actually very limited.

62/70 STRATEGY

A married couple applies for benefits for the partner with the lower income and benefit at age 62, while the higher-earning partner waits until age 70 to apply for benefits. When one partner dies — it doesn't matter which one — the survivor gets to keep the higher benefit. This is also called the FAASF strategy ("file as a spouse first").

DOUBLE DIPPING

This is another strategy for married folks. If you are of full retirement age, you can opt to take your spousal benefit (which would, in most cases, be 50 percent of your spouse's PIA) A good idea is to take the spousal benefit of the partner with the lower-paying full benefit early in order to allow the larger benefit to grow until FRA, or at age 66/67 or 70 to get the bigger benefit later. Let's say the spousal benefit (which has to be specified on the application) would be $1,000 at retirement age 62 and the regular benefit would be $1,200. Normally we think $200 today is worth more than $200 several years from now, but if the person can wait (whether divorced after being married for at least 10 years or widow/widower), delaying taking one's own benefit until age 70 would raise the monthly benefit by a large amount — at least 25 percent. This is the only "raise" you can expect after retirement.

FILE AND SUSPEND

You can file for Social Security benefits and then immediately suspend them (in the "Remarks" section of the application). The higher-earning spouse would do this, with the intent of lifting the suspension when he is 70 and the benefit is much higher. Meanwhile, the spouse can claim either the spousal benefit or his own benefit. The file-and-suspend strategy brings the spousal benefit revenue into the household while still preserving the ability to delay the actual claim until it's worth more in dollar value, and results in a higher survivor payment.

START-OVER STRATEGY

If you are already collecting your Social Security benefits but you have a good stash of savings, you can file to halt your payments, repay all the money you have received from Social Security (with no interest charged for the use of the money), and re-apply at for the higher benefits paid to those aged 66 (if you started at 62) or at 70. Hardly anyone does this despite a fair amount of publicity. Check out Form 521 ("Request for Withdrawal of Application") from the agency's website (SSA.gov). Remember, the amount of increase in the monthly benefit can be 75 percent by taking benefits at the higher age, and the surviving spouse gets to keep the higher amount, too.

Drawbacks include coming up with $100,000 or whatever the cumulative benefits were, tangling with the Social Security Administration for a few months until the amounts get straightened out, and having to pay Medicare separately since, when you stop getting Social Security, you also stop making the Medicare contribution. Be aware that you can do the start-over only once. If you started receiving Social Security at 62, you can start over at 66 but you can't do it again at 70.

Working and Social Security

You can continue to work at your regular job, take a new job, or start a business while collecting Social Security. But to avoid earnings limits, you need to have reached FRA (or be officially disabled). If you are under 66, the current FRA for baby boomers, your earnings limit is $15,120 in 2013. If you earn more than that, $1 dollar is deducted for every $2 you earn over the limit. The deduction is named a "work deduction." Earnings are those from an employer or from self-employment, and do not include bonuses, commissions, severance pay, tips, any other kinds of compensation, investment or rental income, or inheritances. Note that Social Security counts job wages even if you pay Social Security taxes on the wages.

Let's say you had earnings of $20,000. Subtract the earnings limit of $15,129, leaving $4,880 in "excess earnings." Half of that is $2,440 — the amount that will be deducted from your benefits. Unfortunately, the SSA takes it upfront, so that if your monthly payment is $1,200, you would not get any benefit payment in January or February, and your March payment would have the remaining $40 deducted. But in an odd twist of bureaucratic fate, you will get the withheld payments back after you reach FRA. The rules are a little different for the self-employed, who typically do not draw a regular monthly income. In this case, working 45 hours or more in a month is considered "substantial," and will trigger a review. The SSA gets to decide whether to apply an annual or monthly benefit limit.

After you start receiving benefits, in December of each year the SSA will mail to you a notice of the benefit change for the upcoming year due to the cost-of-living increase (1.5 percent in 2014) and the amount of your income that is taxable. To quote the notice directly: "If you were 'full' retirement age (currently age 66) or older throughout the year, you may keep all of your benefits no matter how much you earn. But if you were younger than FRA at any time during the year, there is a limit to how much you can earn before your benefits are reduced.

- If you were younger than full retirement age all year in 2013, the earnings limit was $15,120. We must deduct $1 from your benefits for each $2 you earned over $15,120.

- If you reached full retirement age during 2013, the earnings limit was $40,080. We must deduct $1 from your benefits for each $3 you earned over $40,080 until the month you turned age 66.

- For 2014, "the earnings limit for workers who are younger than full retirement age will be $15,480. The earnings limit for people turning 66 in 2014 will be $41,400." (The earnings limit changes every year.)

Taxing Social Security

Social Security benefits are taxable. Many people are surprised to hear this, because it seems illogical to pay someone a "benefit" funded by one tax only to turn around and collect taxes on the benefit as income. The tax money goes to the Social Security Administration, by the way.

The first 15 percent of your Social Security benefits are tax-free; after that, taxes are applied to the remaining 85 percent. Before looking at the taxable amounts, first you have to calculate something called your "combined income."

Combined Income = Adjusted Gross Income + Nontaxable Interest + Half of SS Benefits (Non-taxable interest is chiefly interest income from municipal bonds.)

Now you compare your combined income to the IRS base amount, which is $25,000 for an individual and $35,000 for a couple filing jointly. Combined income below those thresholds does not trigger a tax on Social Security benefits. But if your combined income exceeds the base amount, here's how it shakes out:

Individuals with a combined income between $25,000 and $34,000: Income tax must be paid on as much as 50 percent of your benefits. With a combined income over $35,000, up to 85 percent of Social Security benefit may be taxable.

Married couples filing jointly with a combined income between $32,000 and $44,000 will be required to pay income tax on as much as 50 percent of benefits. With a combined income over $44,000, up to 85 percent of Social Security benefits may be taxable.

After you start receiving benefits, the SSA will mail you a benefit statement every January showing the amount that you received in the previous year. You can use this statement when doing your taxes. You can either make estimated, quarterly tax payments or have the estimated taxes withheld from your benefits.

If you have a high combined income that subjects your benefits to high taxation, tax lawyers may have ideas for you. Before paying a tax-law expert, use the worksheets in IRS Publication 915, *Social Security and Equivalent Railroad Retirement Benefits*, to compute your taxes. In practice, measures to reduce income to avoid paying taxes on Social Security benefits are thin on the ground, and mostly pertain to other aspects of financial planning, such as switching from IRA to Roth accounts, gifts, estate planning, and real estate.

Social Security Disability Benefit Claims on the Rise

In recent years, the boomer generation (those between 50 and 68) has been cited as the cause of the soaring number of disability benefit claims eating away at the Federal Disability Insurance Trust Fund — fed by a fixed proportion of taxes collected through the Federal Insurance Contributions Act (FICA) and/or the Self-Employment Contributions Act (SECA), which also fund Social Security, Medicare, and Medicaid programs. Media pundits, politicians, and bloggers posit that many of America's unemployed have no plans to return to the workforce, in favor of collecting unemployment, and when those benefits run out, they elect to collect disability benefits, essentially "living on the dole."

Among the unemployed, there are those who were, at one time, being compensated much more handsomely for the same job, or those having to consider low-paying jobs outside of their field of expertise. Disillusioned and feeling that years of hard work hasn't paid off, they see no reason to remain in the workforce. Once the unemployment benefits are discontinued, such individuals find themselves more unemployable than ever, and disabilitiy benefits are sought, often fraudulently — a classic case of a bad apple spoiling the whole cart.

When we consider that those on disability are eligible for Medicare, many blue collar workers stand to gain more on disability than on the job. What's worse is that those on disability aren't included in unemployment statistics, masking the core problem even further.

Conversely, such claims fly in the faces of workers who have invested thirty or more years in blue collar jobs only to find themselves phased out of the workforce — unemployed and unemployable. Jobs that require physical labor, for instance, eventually cause such conditions as severe arthritis and back conditions at the least, compounded by the atrophy that sets in after sitting idle while unemployed, naturally resulting in disability. And considering that boomers over fifty comprise such a large segment of America's population, it's no wonder that disability claims have seen an unusually sharp increase.

Unemployment has not only taken a toll on benefit funds, but has also taken a very human toll, as the rise in mortality rate among the elderly unemployed — especially older men during the initial years of unemployment — has seen a 50 percent increase on the low end, according to *The New York Times* article, "The Human Disaster of Unemployment." An even more disturbing result of this rise in unemployment is an exorbitant rate of suicide among the jobless, a sad but typical product of recession and budgetary austerity measures, not only in the United States, but worldwide.

As the powers that be search for a solution to the unemployment and disability crisis, government seems to be swimming against this current, having extended unemployment benefits eleven times since 2008, with no end in sight. And this classic game of tug-o'-war continues, as one side calls for job creation in the private sector as a solution, and the other contends that extending unemployment even further will put money back into the economy.

How does this affect boomers, not to mention the rest of the population? The Social Security Administration reports that the Disability Trust is due to be completely depleted as of 2016. The Social Security tax payroll has already taken the brunt of this crisis, and such program cuts will continue until we see unemployed Americans, namely boomers 50 and older, returning to the workplace.

Other Aspects of Social Security

Social Security has benefits for minors and spouses under special circumstances. These cases can become incredibly complicated and we will not cover them here. The principle of Social Security addressing poverty is important, though. For example, the spousal benefit of a worker claiming Social Security is 50 percent if the spouse is caring for a child under 16 or a disabled child, even if the spouse is younger than 62, and the benefit rises to 75 percent if the worker dies. Children under 18 are eligible for benefits if their parent is retired, disabled, or deceased. Eligible children are all children — biological, adopted, step, and even dependent adopted grandchildren. A big family can collect up to 180 percent of a worker's Social Security benefit. If you have a complicated family situation, be aware that Social Security workers who answer the phones are not allowed to give you advice, but can provide the appropriate information if you know the right questions to ask.

Finally, the Social Security Death Benefit is a flat, lump-sum of $255 per Social Security beneficiary. You must file within two years of the death to collect. Visit SSA.gov for more information.

Remember to heed the following, simple "do's and don'ts" when considering retirement and your Social Security benefit:

DaVINCI DO'S

- As you near retirement, always keep in mind that Social Security is not meant as a sole means of income, but as a supplement to your savings. Even at the eleventh hour, it's never too late to begin saving and researching alternate plans.

- If you're not receiving an annual statement of scheduled Social Security benefits, go to SSA.gov/estimator for a breakdown of your earnings history and estimated future benefit.

- Remember that divorced spouses can claim essentially the same benefits as current spouses if the marriage lasted at least ten years and the divorced claimant is currently unmarried.

DaVINCI DON'TS

- Everyone's situation varies at least a little, and some are very complex. Don't take a well-meaning neighbor or friend's advice when it comes to your Social Security benefit filing strategy. For detailed advice, an excellent resource to consult is former Social Security Administrator Andy Landis' book, *Social Security, The Inside Story*. And if you don't manage to get your hands on the book, Landis has this basic pearl of wisdom to offer: "The bottom line is that if you just want the most dollars from SSA and expect to live past age 78, file at 66, not 62."

- Don't forget that if you are collecting benefits and still working, if you are under the age of 66 (the current Full Retirement Age) you are subject to an earnings limit. If you go over that limit, $1 of every $2 earned will be collected. The limit changes each year.

- Don't hesitate to consult with Social Security representatives for basic questions and inquiries between the hours of 7 a.m. and 7 p.m., Monday through Friday, at (800) 772-1213, (800) 325-0778 (TTY). There is also have a 24-hour, automated line with recorded information: (800)772-1213.

A Place to Call Home in Your Golden Years

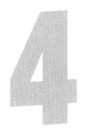

JUST ABOUT EVERYBODY would like to stay in his own home and not have to shift to assisted living, let alone the dreaded nursing home. We think of the United States as having a very mobile population, but the inclination to move actually peaks in the early 20s, and falls off sharply at about 50–55, where it stays relatively flat. According to the Research Institute for Housing America (RIHA), the very oldest have a small propensity to move.

It's tough to draw the distinction between housing and real estate. Housing is literally having a roof over your head and an address where you get mail, while real estate can be viewed as a financial asset as well as a physical one. If you have owned your home for a long time and paid off your mortgage or nearly paid it off, it is correct to think of your house as one of your financial assets — possibly your biggest one. The thought of cashing it in is terrifying, as it should be — you would be swapping home and housing for mere money.

That's why selling your house as a strategy to get the funds for a move to smaller, cheaper quarters or assisted living may be a good strategy — but only if you are really sure about the conditions. Scammers abound, ringing your doorbell claiming to be agents with contracts from buyers, when really they just want to get your house at below-market cost and flip it. The "agent" pressures you to sign the contract. Some real estate experts advise that you put the house along with other assets in a trust so that any sale has to be signed by the trustee, too.

Another cash-out strategy is the reverse mortgage, advertised on TV by popular actors. Reverse mortgages could serve as a very viable alternative for the appropriate candidate, but such mortgages became so controversial over the past few years that the Federal Trade Commission stepped in to offer guidance and a place to report abuse. If you're considering a reverse mortgage, protect yourself from potential fraud by visiting Consumer.FTC.gov/articles/0192-reverse-mortgages.

If you are a renter, you are protected against age discrimination by the federal Fair Housing Act of 1968 and the federal Fair Housing Act Amendments of 1988, but landlords can jack up your rent to unacceptable levels in order to get you out. Some cities and states offer those over 62 or 65 some protection from rent increases, although you have to be willing to deal with state agencies and possibly go to court. This is no fun when you are 75, and sometimes not feasible when you are 85.

Homeownership vs "Real Estate"

Everyone has a real estate story to tell by the time they near retirement. For most of the early boomers, it's a great tale of wealth accumulation, beginning with the nostalgia of buying the first home. Some were lucky enough to buy that first house and stay in it through most of their adult lives, paying off the mortgage long ago. For still others, moving up the career ladder, marrying, and starting a family has gone hand in hand with the decision to sell a smaller home and move up to newer, spacious, and more valuable homes. Along the way, many have built a sizeable nest egg simply by owning the home they lived in.

Early- to middle-boomers, in particular those 65 years of age and older, have been the most successful of all US age-groups in achieving high ownership rates: Over 80 percent own their own homes, based on findings by RHIA. Even the Great Recession didn't put a dent in this age group's ownership rates; though there was a slight decline from 2004 to 2008, it has since recovered. With most of the older group having paid off mortgages, built up equity that didn't completely disappear in the downturn, and receiving a steady, inflation-adjusted, Social Security income, early boomers were relatively immune from the shocks of the last decade.

Younger boomers (those under 65), and the generations of boomers' children in their 30s and 40s, took the biggest hit during the past recession. Their rates of ownership have declined, representing the loss of homes in the midst of unstable job markets. Many have inadequate incomes for the cost of renting (let alone owning) in unaffordable, coastal urban markets like New York, San Francisco, and Los Angeles. Lending standards have been tightened time and again to prevent a repeat of the overly-lax environment that led to many loan defaults and foreclosures. As a result, younger families with stagnant or declining real incomes will have to wait longer to save enough to enter the housing ownership market, if at all.

Ownership rates are lower still among those with less than a college education. Many of those working class and immigrant families who entered the ownership ranks for the first time after being renters have simply been returned to the rental marketplace; their landlords may now be hedge funds and other institutions, which have been major buyers of foreclosed homes throughout the country, paying cash and frequently acquiring large groups of homes in bulk purchases. As an article on Minnesota's MinnPost.com revealed in its December 3, 2013, issue, the globe's largest private equity firm, Blackstone Group, had spent $7.5 billion on 40,000 properties in 14 housing markets for its Invitation Homes partnership, making it the largest landlord of single-family houses in several cities. And based on a recent South Florida *Sun Sentinel* article, the firm is still at it, having purchased 430 properties between January and May of 2014 in Palm Beach County alone — more than double that of the same period in 2013.

But for all its recent trials and tribulations, home ownership has been the backbone of the economy and the largest store of personal wealth in the post-World War II era. Equity in the family home is by far the largest personal asset of American households: for

Age	Equity-to-Annual Income Ratio
TABLE 4-1: MEDIAN HOUSING EQUITY-TO-INCOME RATIO	
Ages 90 +	5.07:1
Ages 85-89	4.33:1
Ages 80-84	4.08:1
Ages 75-79	3.51:1
Ages 70-74	3.00:1
Ages 65-69	2.33:1
Ages 60-64	1.83:1
Ages 55-59	1.42:1

Source: The Research Institute for Housing America, A Profile of Housing and Health Among Older Americans, http://www.housingamerica.org/RIHA/RIHA/Publications/86310_13205_RIHA_Senior_Housing_Paper.pdf

middle to late boomers, it represents 50 percent of their personal wealth, at a median amount of $125,000.

In Table 4-1, the translated data findings from The Research Institute for Housing America show that the overall housing equity ratio for older Americans was 2.35 times their annual income. Considering their calculation of a 2013 median equity of $125,000 and a median annual income (from all sources) of $50,583, these figures are modest in view of the need for funding a long retirement.

Most boomers who saved and paid down their mortgages will still need the use of their homes and the ability to tap the resource of that equity as they age.

The importance of the home's equity value increases with advancing age and declining income, as the November 2013 study from the Research Institute for Housing America shows. What is reflected in the equity-to-income ratios might contain some good news in that the family home will retain some store of value if you can just stay in it. But the clearly increasing ratio more likely underscores the fact that after age 65, total earned income will be declining as you get older.

Cashing-Out

So, how do we juggle the retention of value in the savings vehicle we know best — homeownership — with the increasing need to supplement income? The thought of cashing in the family home is terrifying, as it should be; it has been your safe haven — your tangible nest egg as well as your nesting-place.

One safe fallback many people have kept in their pocket is having, but not tapping into, a home equity line of credit, referred to in the trade as a HELOC. This was designed to let homeowners with sufficient equity draw bits out here and there, rather than take out a second mortgage. The idea here is that if there were a major emergency like a medical crisis where insurance is not sufficient, you could write a check against the line, have use of the funds, and have the goal of paying it back quickly without building up too much interest expense.

But in the last decade, the idea of the homeowner having the kind of line-of-credit flexibility once only given to business customers got out of control. Marketing by banks grew less cautious; soon mortgage brokers and loan officers began using the angle of selling equity lines (as opposed to second mortgages) to consumers so that they could draw on it at a low rate in order to pay off high-interest debts like installment loans and credit cards. The trouble was that people who had lots of credit card debt that they rolled into home equity weren' t really in a position to pay back the equity line as quickly as was hoped.

The worst abuse came as lenders drove for more loan product to resell in the marketplace. Don't have a sufficient down payment? Now you could borrow against equity in the home before you even took ownership, in order to squeeze into a house at the top of the hot 2005-2006 market peak, bringing us products requiring no down payment or little-to-no documentation, like the 80/20 loan, the No-Doc loan, the NINA (no income/no asset), the SISA (stated income/stated asset), and so on . . .

We know how these stories ended. With leverage and mortgage payments increasing just as large sections of the population lost jobs and income, real estate markets took their sharpest dive since the Great Depression.

When the dust settled, inevitably foreclosures proliferated. The reason we revisit this history is to explain the paradox of what has happened to both older and younger people who stayed in their houses, and didn't take out extravagant loans. These folks saw the home equity account, barely used, as an insurance policy for future emergencies as originally intended.

So what happened? By the end of the crisis, many of the well-managed but untapped credit resources were quickly drawn back by the banks. If a credit line hadn't been used, then it could get cancelled. If a small amount was still on account, then the bank might trim back the credit line to perhaps half of the unused amount.

As banks reverted to strict underwriting guidelines in order to comply with new responsible-lending procedures (ironically put in place by the same regulators who allowed financiers to run amuck and subsequently bailed them out), it has become harder and harder for responsible borrowers and those rebuilding credit to qualify under the current standards. Lenders now require stricter, verifiable debt-to-income and loan-to-value ratios. If your loan is not processed within a month's time or more, it's possible that you'll be submitting the same documentation a second, and perhaps even a third time. Also, your final interest rate is now much more dependent on a credit score higher than the once-standard, 620 minimum.

In this environment, seniors seeking to obtain credit encounter an especially harsh challenge. What is most important is that you maintain good, low-cost credit by taking advantage of your peak in earnings before retirement. It must also be accompanied by the discipline of not using that credit unless it makes sense in your financial plan.

Reverse Mortgages

Another loan product that came under considerable scrutiny during the recent mortgage loan debacle is the reverse mortgage — known as the Home Equity Conversion Mortgage (HECM) by the FHA — which is specifically marketed toward the elderly and their families. Like any other loan product, when marketed earnestly and to the appropriate candidate, the reverse mortgage could be a viable solution for a specific segment of the population.

HOW DO REVERSE MORTGAGES WORK?

As the term implies, instead of making monthly mortgage payments, you can elect to receive monthly payments from the existing equity in your home. In order to qualify, among other requirements, you must either own the home outright or have an existing mortgage small enough to be paid off with the proceeds of the reverse mortgage at closing and still have enough remaining equity to generate a monthly payment that is practical.

Because reverse mortgages are designed for long-term payments to last until your death, like an annuity, the issuer will structure the payment size based on the age of the youngest owner. If you take out a reverse mortgage at the minimum allowable age of 62, the payments you will receive will be much smaller than if you start when you are 80, for example.

The reverse mortgage was originally designed to allow the owner to retain his or her home while receiving funds to supplement income for, ostensibly, expenses that come in later life. These are not loans to be used for trips to Europe and monthly groceries. This distinction is important: These loans are ideally designed to pay for end-of-life care when all other resources have been tapped.

Like other non-conventional loan products, the reverse mortgage is not ideal for the typical retiree. While a qualified borrower can be as young as 62, getting a recommendation at that age to consider this type of loan should be a red flag. Starting the loan at 62 will mean that the payments must stretch over your "remaining life," which these days could be much longer than in the past — it could be 30 more years. Stretch it out, and the actual monthly income generated by the mortgage for you to use will be that much more modest.

The reverse mortgage loan itself is more complex to structure and administer, which means, understandably, it will be more expensive than the traditional mortgage. That higher interest rate is churning away at a declining balance of home equity.

Another factor to consider is that even though the reverse mortgage is providing income, the owner must still maintain the home and pay property taxes. Unfortunately, the way reverse mortgages were set up, there was no mechanism for the banks to monitor whether borrowers had the physical and financial resources for the upkeep of their homes. For this reason, the major lenders — Wells Fargo, Bank of America, and MetLife — exited this market in 2011 and 2012 citing losses and Fed-oversight concerns, indicating that about 4 to 5 percent of these loans were already in default on one or both items.

In the case of default, or where the equity is exhausted by a drastic market drop years down the road, a forced sale could be triggered, perhaps at the most inconvenient time of life for this to

REVERSE MORTGAGE DO'S AND DON'TS:

Do as much research as possible, being sure to choose an FHA approved lender if you do decide that a reverse mortgage is for you.

Do be sure to gather and calculate property tax figures, association fees, homeowner's and flood/windstorm insurance premiums, and utilities before pursuing counseling.

Do take into consideration that this loan is meant for a borrower whose home is intended to be their principal residence, and if the borrow needs to move out of the home (and into assisted living, for instance), or becomes deceased, the loan will come due.

Don't trust the opinion of the Henry Winkler, Robert Wagner, or any other salesperson, neighbor, or friend when considering this loan. Instead, take advantage of FHA mortgage counseling to assess your own, individual situation before making a decision to go forward with any home loan.

Don't forget that these loans carry with them high origination fees, as well as an up-front mortgage insurance premium and other fees, so closing costs will be unusually higher than a conventional loan.

Don't consider a reverse mortgage unless you've exhausted all other savings and assets first.

happen. Most heirs are usually not in a position to quickly cover the loan when it is called in due to the default or the death of the holder. Another result to consider: Taking out a reverse mortgage, especially over a long period, will almost certainly lead to the sale of the family home, whether you like it or not. Your children will probably not be able to inherit the home if this is the major item in your estate.

If you are considering a reverse mortgage, the best place to start is the US Department of Housing and Urban Development (HUD), which now requires you to undergo mortgage counseling with an FHA approved HECM counselor. For details, you can visit Portal.HUD.gov/hudportal/HUD?src=/program_offices/housing/sfh/hecm/hecmabou, or call (800) 569-4287 to speak with a counselor.

A Family Affair

While many of us, for a variety of reasons, live far from loved ones, for others, the family unit is central to daily life. As mentioned in Chapter 2, some have purchased or built homes with attached in-law quarters, intending to house aging parents or to someday occupy it themselves. In times of economic hardship, or simply to play an active role in the lives of children and grandchildren, a viable solution to retirement housing is to pool resources and share expenses with family. For homes that are lacking in accommodations, perhaps a remodel or addition is an option, which can be funded by the additional household income and/or savings while increasing the home's value.

Multigenerational households are the norm in many cultures outside of the United States, and are beneficial not only from an economic perspective, but provide a solid support system, as well as staving off loneliness and isolation that could lead to depression. For the senior members of the household, sharing daily activities like preparing dinner with your daughter or reading a book to your grandchild can actually prolong the onset of senility, while making for a richer life and deeper, overall sense of well-being.

Downsizing

The majority of retirees plan to stay close to friends and family — perhaps even in the same town.

But the family home in which you raised your kids may simply be too big to maintain, or it just makes empty-nest syndrome all that more apparent to you. If you're among the many who just don't have enough saved, it might be a consideration that some of that equity is better used to downsize now and have more assets available as part of retirement savings.

Still others see their own parents or older friends develop mobility issues and realize their three-level, hillside-view home will become less practical in ten or twenty years. In the hilly terrain of California, having a "level-in" or large, single story home already commands a premium from affluent boomers.

Many people who have not dealt with moving or selling over the years still think selling a house requires rolling the proceeds over into the next one for tax purposes, or that the capital gains exemption is a one-time benefit for those over 55.

Guess what? The capital-gains rule on owner-occupied homes changed in the 1990s, and a very generous exemption from capital gains was phased in. Profits, not sales prices, of $250,000 for singles and $500,000 for couples are capital gains-exempt for those who have occupied their home for two out of the last five years of ownership. That amount of profit would make the sale of most boomers' homes tax-free. Since there are new attempts to nibble away at this benefit, it might be prudent to take advantage of this rule before it is reduced or phased out.

Managing the Real Estate Broker

If you have decided it's time to sell the family home, there comes the matter of dealing with the transaction. And if you haven't dealt with a real estate agent in many years, here are some suggestions:

You probably shouldn't do this yourself. Hiring an agent will cost around 5 to 6 percent of the sales proceeds, but your home should have the most exposure to the marketplace through the local Multiple Listing Service (MLS). Having an intermediary is a good thing for such an important transaction, especially given the emotional attachment involved — you may instantly dislike the people who come to "take" your house. However, there are some instances where selling "by owner" could work: if you have bought and sold frequently and know the pitfalls; if you live in a state where a title company/attorney can handle all the legal and contractual requirements at a modest cost; and if you already have a known and ready buyer or the market in your area is so hot that just putting a for sale sign in your yard will generate calls, you may save some money. However, the stress factor and the potential ability of a good agent to get your home exposure and sell it for more, beyond what their commission would cover, are good arguments for hiring a realtor.

If possible, work with an SRES certified agent. The Seniors Real Estate Specialists Council of the National Association of Realtors offers an intensive educational program, awarding successful participants an SRES certification. Whether buying or selling, SRES designated real estate agents are trained to address the needs of those aged 50 and over. Newly retired individuals and seniors occupy a completely different market than, say, a couple buying their first home. SRES agents are adept at catering to the needs of the boomer generation in such areas as selling the family home, downsizing, relocating, or offering senior-friendly financing/refinancing options.

The SRES focuses on helping to mitigate the stress associated with shedding a lifetime of accumulated belongings, as well as dealing with the sale of homes that haven't been updated for quite some time. When it comes to purchasing, they can help you select a home that will fulfill your current and future needs, such as choosing a floor plan that will accommodate a caregiver down the road, if need be. Their training also enables them to offer invaluable

advice in areas such as leveraging investments and reverse mortgages, steering you away from common financial mistakes as well
as scams. Consult SeniorsRealestate.com/50-real-estate-resources
to find an SRES specialist, or call (800) 500-4564.

**The name you see most often is not always the best agent
for you.** Heavily advertised agents are, to be sure, busy, aggressive, and colorful personalities. But they may tend to place their
own interests above yours; their success is measured by crank-
ing toward goals of quick, numerous, and profitable transactions
without regard for your personal situation. They will use a lot of
"success seminar" jargon, and set limits with you about how they
work in order to control how you communicate with each other,
again, based on a learned formula rather than on a more human,
personal level.

Beware the "team." Top producers often develop a system of
drawing in clients with their dynamic style and aura of success.
Then suddenly, the boring stuff, like filling out forms, showing
your house, and marketing it are delegated to the junior members
who are learning the craft, not quite ready to strike out on their
own. They get to practice on you.

Look for a good background and accessible references. Real
estate draws all kinds of people — a cross section of society. It's
often a positive, late-career choice (the current median age of realtors nationally is 56) for people who are tired of the corporate
world, but also a way station for those not wishing to look unemployed during a downturn. The basic real estate licensing requirements in most states can be completed in a matter of a couple of
weekends. So we might have your probable largest single financial
transaction, when your home is sold or bought, handled by someone who requires fewer hours of training and education to be let
loose on the public than your neighborhood barber at Supercuts.
The job is not uncomplicated, but because states and realtor professional organizations benefit from the fees generated by a vast
number of inactive or barely active licensees, they haven't raised
the barriers to entry. On the other hand, you may luck out and get
an experienced former teacher, lawyer, or psychologist as a realtor.

**Your aunt's best friend's daughter is probably not going to
be the best choice.** After the description of the limited training
a realtor might have, you don't wait to give your friend's relative

a break and be a guinea pig if they are brand-new in the industry. Rely on friends' experiences with a realtor in specific and recent transactions from start to finish, not whether they socialize with them; rely on the former as a gauge of professional ability, as word-of-mouth is still the best and most reliable form of advertisement. An experienced realtor should know the area and market well, help you with tough negotiations, and be your advocate. If you don't sense those capabilities in the realtor you're considering, keep looking.

Interview more than one realtor before hiring. Most realtors would like to presume they are working for you exclusively in the first five minutes after meeting you, unless you say otherwise. So do tell them you're interviewing a few people. Structure it like a search, but keep it realistic. Telling someone you're interviewing ten of their peers is a signal you're going to be a difficult client; it may make you lose the chance for a good fit, because busy but competent agents won't bother to participate. Look at the type of business they're doing online — are they listing or selling houses in your neighborhood that are similar to yours? Did the listings sell for a good price in a reasonable amount of time? Ask for references from clients who are willing to speak to you, especially if you don't know anyone who's had direct experience with them. Once you have the right match, stick with them and don't work with more than one. You can always switch if doesn't work out, depending on the timing of your listing contract.

Negotiating the commission. You can get a good read on your realtor by how he deals with the issue of the commission. If he tells you the commission is "x" percent, it's an attempt to gloss it over. If you start to negotiate, you may hear a canned speech about "why I charge three percent" that includes the idea that the realtor has to get paid a lot to negotiate hard on your behalf later. This may sound reasonable, but be aware that sticking to a fixed commission is part of their training to get you to cave. On the other hand, drive the commission too low, and you remember the old cliché: You only get what you pay for. There may be less advertising and marketing for your listing because you're not paying the going rate, and a marketplace of realtors who will effectively boycott your listing because they feel they're not going to get paid enough.

Renting vs. Buying

While the most boomers are homeowners, some may transition into rental housing to try out their next steps, such as downsizing, moving closer to family or moving to an entirely new place. An increasing number of younger boomers will have been renters through much of their lives. A new Harvard study shows that growth in the rental population among those heading into retirement ages went up 4 to 6 percent during the period 2009-2013, reflecting financial distress among the younger boomers.

Generally speaking, there is a great variation in metro areas when considering rental markets. Rental rates are highest in cities of the Northeast, where, based on research performed by Harvard University's Joint Center for Housing Studies, more than 60 percent of households rent, compared with 45–50 percent in other regions. About a quarter of households rent in suburban and non-metropolitan areas in most parts of the country, although rates in these areas exceed 30 percent in the West.

Those who occupy a low-priced, rent-controlled apartment in an otherwise expensive location like Manhattan, San Francisco, or Santa Monica would not be motivated to buy anytime soon, but even market rents in those areas tend to be lower than the cost of owning, depending on salary levels, mortgage rates, and price trends. Consequently, the largest cities with the highest proportion of renters are New York (72 percent); Boston (68 percent); Los Angeles (66 percent) and San Francisco (64 percent), as reported by ZipAtlas.com.

Affordability also relates to the ability to purchase a home and make mortgage payments based on the salaries available in a local job market. Generally, where real estate prices are high, average or median salaries may be proportionately higher, as in the major, coastal metro areas. So while the aforementioned cities would be automatically expected to come in low on the affordability list, there are others where more moderately priced homes can be less "affordable."

For example, some high-priced resort and retirement areas, especially with world-class beach or ski resorts, depend on those who bring established wealth to live there and fuel the local real estate market. Those dependent on the local, salaried economy for a living, and even those making more than a local median salary may be priced out of their own market. Indeed, there is an increasing trend of rental "cost burden" in many parts of the United States. As rents increased and incomes have decreased, more than 28 percent of renters are paying more than 50 percent of their income for housing.

TABLE 4-2: WHERE BUYING A HOME IS A TOUGHER CALL

US Metro	Cost of Buying vs. Renting (%), Summer 2013	Cost of Buying vs. Renting (%), Summer 2012	Mortgage Rate Tipping Point When Renting Becomes Cheaper Than Buying, Summer 2013
San Jose, CA	-4%	-31%	5.2%
San Francisco, CA	-9%	-28%	5.7%
Honolulu, HI	-10%	-24%	5.8%
Orange County, CA	-20%	-34%	7.0%
New York, NY-NJ	-21%	-31%	7.5%
San Diego, CA	-21%	-34%	7.3%
Los Angeles, CA	-21%	-32%	7.3%
Ventura County, CA	-22%	-33%	7.5%
Oakland, CA	-23%	-43%	7.5%
Sacramento, CA	-26%	-39%	8.2%

Source: http://www.trulia.com/trends/2013/09/rent-vs-buy-summer-2013/

TABLE 4-3: WHERE BUYING A HOME IS A NO-BRAINER

US Metro	Cost of Buying vs. Renting (%), Summer 2013	Cost of Buying vs. Renting (%), Summer 2012	Mortgage Rate Tipping Point When Renting Becomes Cheaper Than Buying, Summer 2013
Detroit, MI	-65%	-70%	32.8%
Gary, IN	-58%	-63%	20.6%
Memphis, TN-MS-AR	-55%	-61%	19.0%
Cleveland, OH	-54%	-60%	20.0%
Kansas City, MO-KS	-53%	-57%	18.0%
Warren-Troy-Farmington Hills, MI	-53%	-61%	18.4%
Dayton, OH	-53%	-61%	19.5%
Grand Rapids, MI	-52%	-57%	17.7%
West Palm Beach, FL	-52%	-59%	17.1%
Akron, OH	-51%	-55%	18.2%

Source: http://www.trulia.com/trends/2013/09/rent-vs-buy-summer-2013/

Trulia.com measured the changes in affordability brought about by shifts in prices and rates in its 2013 survey. It found that mortgage rate increases will make the most significant changes in an area's affordability, using the assumption of a 20 percent down payment, 4.8 percent interest rate, and often a prepayment penalty. As the costs and prices vary over time, they calculated a tipping point at which more expensive mortgages will send that area into a more favored environment for renting.

You may have noticed that the mortgage interest tax deduction is excluded from the comparison of the various metro areas with consideration to buying vs renting. The reason? While just 33 percent of all taxpayers itemize, using the mortgage interest deduction will eliminate any benefit to renting in even the most expensive markets. In Trulia's survey, all the metro areas reviewed proved to favor home ownership when federal tax considerations were added to the comparison.

Both Trulia.com and the NYTimes.com offer tools to use one's own measurements, such as rental increases, purchase holding periods, and real estate price trends to calculate whether it makes sense to buy or rent. Google "Trulia rent vs. buy" and "NYTimes rent vs. buy."

Boomer Mobility

While there are many fantasies to consider about where to go and what to do in retirement, the fact remains that most people will stay close to their original homes, families, and friends. An Urban Institute study of 2010 Census Bureau data indicates that only 1.6 percent of retirees between the ages of 55 and 65 plan to move across state lines.

With respect to those hailing from the Midwest and Northeast, though the migration patterns have shifted from Florida to some other eastern-seaboard destinations in recent years, there are still those looking to relocate to the Sunshine State in order to gain some tax relief. What New Yorker, Illinoisan, or Pennsylvanian wouldn't, considering that Florida boasts no individual income tax, no inheritance tax, nor an estate tax. Folks escaping California's high tax burden are most likely to choose Arizona or Texas. Big property stocks left over from the real estate "boom and bust" combined with significantly lower property taxes in the levy-friendly states offer further impetus to flee.

As opposed to those seeking refuge from the taxman, many have decided against balmy Florida in favor of a locale that offered some warmth, accompanied by a gentle, four-season climate. Upon leaving Florida, instead of returning to their relatives in the Northeast or Midwest, many stopped in some attractive parts of Georgia and the Carolinas — and were sold. The Brookings Institution found that more and more late boomers have these areas in mind as first, target moving destinations, with places like Raleigh/Durham, Wilmington, Asheville, and Myrtle Beach showing tremendous growth in the 65+ population.

Other than proximity to friends and family as the major determinant of where older and younger boomers will choose to live, when polled on actual preferences in 2012 by Mason-Dixon Polling & Research, the most important factors in considering relocation are:

- Having top-quality healthcare facilities nearby (96%)

- Affordable housing (92%)

- Warm climate (85.5%), "but a strong plurality wants the warm summers to be paired with a few cooler months"

- Low local taxes (81%)

- Affordable recreational opportunities and strong local elder care services (80%)

- A mid-sized city or small town (70%)

- Arts and cultural opportunities (75%)

- Proximity to beaches or ocean (60%)

- Life-long learning opportunities (50%)

- Community that welcomes diversity (50%)

- University nearby (40%)

While most people will agree these are all positive factors for any place to live, the ideal combination in a single "best place" is elusive. People's tastes and interests about where they live are widely different. Some people hate the beach, and some love the mountains. Others love the wide open spaces, and still others aren't going to give up bustling, culturally-vibrant city life.

The many articles and click-through lists online are going to favor the demographic polled when narrowing down the "best" option. Pay attention to the criteria on which they're ranking cities. Remember some of these lists are created more for fun and publicity — and they want to improve that website's click-through statistics when you go through their lists page by page.

There are some more serious attempts to help you rank your best places, though. The annual *Money Magazine* "Best Places" issues are a good starting point. They can't have the same best places every year, so even the back issues can be relevant for capturing the well-rounded flavor of a place to live.

Other sites, like BestCities.net, CreativeClass.com/whos_your_city, and Kiplinger.com let you construct a list of recommended cities based on your preferences. Once you have a handful of potential cities/towns, one interesting site with lively discussions about the good and bad — warts and all — on living almost anywhere is City-Data.com.

If there are very specific factors that are important to you in your search, there are additional comparison tools available online, such as Outflux.com for climate data and AreaVibes.com for crime-rate comparisons.

Once you've narrowed down your target city, a good idea, if possible, is to visit more than once, at different times of year. Even more specifically, when you've decided on a neighborhood, visit at different times of day. A great way to get a feel for your new neighbors would be to visit the nearest food/grocery store. Other factors to consider are access to local transportation and proximity to a major airport.

As previously discussed, taxes are a huge deal maker or breaker, especially if you're looking for some relief in taxation as part of the retirement relocation. It's not a straightforward comparison. To break the bad news to you: There is no single, totally tax-free haven among the US states. And no matter where you go — even to a place you thought had low taxes — you'll typically end up paying more for something.

There are seven states that have *no state income tax*:

1. Alaska
2. Florida

3. Nevada

4. South Dakota

5. Texas

6. Washington

7. Wyoming

And these five states have *no sales taxes*:

1. Alaska

2. Delaware

3. New Hampshire

4. Oregon

5. Montana

But where the state tax authority giveth, the local assessor might also taketh away. States try to make up for lack of income tax revenue elsewhere, whether with sales tax, property tax, or gas tax. CNN has a good visual chart to show the relationship of property tax dollar amounts versus actual property tax percentage rates: Money.CNN.com/interactive/real-estate/property-tax.

Hidden in some of the reasonably priced real estate and no-income-tax environment of Texas are some of the highest property tax rates in the country, right behind the more notorious New Jersey.

While the dollar amounts of taxes paid on California real estate holdings are astronomical because of the high values, the actual percentage is closer to the national median. But concealed in the otherwise high-tax environment of California are some extraordinary tax breaks that can keep seniors hanging on tight to their property well beyond retirement. Proposition 13 froze assessments and tax rates for those who were in their homes in 1978, increasing only at one percent a year in assessed value, even if the market went up much higher, which it did. Many early boomers who live in affluent areas bought their homes for perhaps $100,000, which was a tidy sum in 1978. They might now still pay about $1,500 per year in property tax, with no fear it might shoot up dramatically from there.

A young couple buying into the same neighborhood might now pay almost $1 million for what is a nice, but not extravagant home on the same street. Because the rates are set based on the current market, the younger couple now pays $15,000 a year tax for essentially the same house as the elderly neighbor who is taxed at $1,500. Additional laws now allow that same elderly owner, rather than being trapped in the big house with low taxes, the option to downsize to a less expensive home in the same county or a limited number of other California counties, and take that same low tax bill with them to the next property. The inequities are apparent, making this law a hot-button issue of California politics.

In states with widely varying property tax rates, it may be just a matter of making the downsizing decision to move to another neighborhood or township where you don't pay as high a rate, because now the quality of the local school system is not important to you.

The lesson here is if a location lands on your list of favorite targets, do some investigation into the peculiarities of not just the state, but also the locality's tax issues. You may not need a tax haven if your state doesn't tax social security or pension income and that's your main source of income. Some will tax interest and dividend income differently. One town with excellent schools, which you no longer need to use, could have a neighboring tax district with much lower rates, for example. This type of significant variation in property tax from town to town is more common in the Northeastern states.

TABLE 4-4: SEVEN STATES WITH NO INCOME TAX (BUT CHECK PROPERTY TAXES AND SALES TAXES AS THE OFFSET)

State	Sales	Property	Estate	Other
Alaska	1-7% (local only)	Over 65 exempt on first $150,000	No	Funding from sale and taxes on oil
Florida	6% + local	Up to $50,000 homestead exemption	No	
Nevada	6.85% + local	Yes	No	Funding from taxes on gambling
South Dakota	4% + local	Some property tax relief for retirees	No	
Texas	6.25% + local	Over 65 some exemption	No	2% fireworks tax
Washington	6.5% + local	Over 65 some exemption	No	
Wyoming	4% + local	9.5%, some exemption for over 65	No	

Source: Respective state's department of revenue websites

A telling survey of the total tax burdens of many US metro areas, including scenarios for income levels, is published annually by the chief financial officer of the District of Columbia. Some interesting names appear on their estimates. With the highest combined, total major tax burden for a family of three, the top five most highly-taxed cities are:

1. Bridgeport, Connecticut
2. Philadelphia, Pennsylvania
3. Columbus, Ohio
4. Newark, New Jersey
5. Louisville, Kentucky

States with the overall highest tax burden are:

1. New York
2. New Jersey
3. Connecticut
4. Wisconsin
5. California

Cities with the overall lowest tax burden are:

1. Cheyenne, Wyoming
2. Anchorage, Alaska
3. Jacksonville, Florida
4. Memphis, Tennessee
5. Houston, Texas

States with the overall lowest tax burden are:

1. Alaska
2. South Dakota
3. Tennessee
4. Louisiana
5. Wyoming

On Retiring Abroad

After reading about the type of savings you need and the prospects for a tighter budget in retirement years, some people glibly state: "If I have to live on Social Security alone, I'll just move abroad." At least a half-million retirees have actually done so — some to great satisfaction and others to disillusionment. Several million have responded affirmatively when polled as to whether they'd consider retiring outside of the United States in the future. To be sure, there are some economies where most of the cost-of-living items, in addition to housing, are significantly cheaper than in the United States. There are many sites dedicated to selling you information about an overseas retirement where there are no problems — you live like a king and are waited on hand and foot by the locals, all for a fraction of your monthly pension. Take these sales pitches with a grain of salt.

While there are many variables that go into the ability to adapt as an expatriate, probably the worst-equipped candidates would be those whose primary motivation is economic distress. With very little experience traveling abroad, let alone living abroad, a retiree who is strictly English-speaking and whose last encounter with a foreign language was a dismal high school course will often find many things more stressful in this new environment than the one left behind.

Aside from those who may have a non-US partner or some other type of existing affinity for a foreign country, not to mention those whose budget can allow for part-time or full-time retirement living in a higher-cost country like Italy or France, there are some options becoming more palatable to the American retiree. Mexico comes to mind first, as it is the closest neighbor and offers many levels of budget living.

Just as a Briton retiring to France, an American retiring to Mexico will have easier access back home for family visits and emergencies in terms of time and cost than either will if retiring to Fiji, for instance. Retirement communities are developing in the usual beach-resort areas popular with American and Canadian travelers: Cabo San Lucas, Loreto, and La Paz on the Baja Peninsula; and Puerto Vallarta, Cancun, and Playa del Carmen on the Yucatan Peninsula. Those who are less interested in beach environments have built large expat communities in picturesque, inland areas like Lake Chapala near Guadalajara and San Miguel de Allende.

Other popular destinations are Panama, Costa Rica, and Belize. Costa Rica was the first country to offer a *pensionado*, or "retiree" visa to Americans that included big tax breaks and discounts on some expenses, although these have mostly been discontinued today. USNews.com reports that "Costa Rica has also become more expensive, both as a place to live and as a place to own a home. For these reasons, while Costa Rica is perhaps the world's most well known overseas retirement haven, it no longer qualifies as one of the best."

Every year, *Forbes* magazine publishes a list of top retirement destinations abroad. The 2014 version showcases the top 15 countries:

1. Panama
2. Ecuador
3. Malaysia
4. Costa Rica
5. Spain
6. Colombia
7. Mexico
8. Malta
9. Uruguay
10. Thailand
11. Ireland
12. New Zealand
13. Nicaragua
14. Italy
15. Portugal

You can find many other articles about retiring abroad from scores of reliable publications, but remember, the reasons why a city or country is advertised as a "good" place to retire may not apply to your situation. In other words, the information is promotional. But for a good fantasy afternoon, check out LiveAndInvestOverseas.com. Finally, the *Huffington Post* published a story on the "6 Places You Can Retire on $1250 A Month Or Less," complete with the cost of rent, utilities, etc., and the list includes:

- Cebu, Philippines
- Chiang Mai, Thailand
- Cuenca, Ecuador
- Granada, Nicaragua
- Hoi An, Vietnam
- Medellin, Colombia

So You're Determined to Take The Plunge

Now that you've taken an honest and searching inventory of your reasons to relocate, have narrowed down your potential relocation destination(s), and still believe that retiring abroad is, in fact, a conceivable and viable option for you, it's time to do the real work.

REAL ESTATE/HOUSING

If you surf the net for real estate abroad, you'll see ad after ad (often disguised as articles) urging you to buy in this location or that, many times at astronomically low prices.

Sales scams can range from the same property being sold multiple times, to developers raising the final sales price after construction is complete, claiming the price-hike was due to "unforeseen costs" — and keeping your sizeable down payment if you back out.

Other problems an unsuspecting foreign consumer may encounter deal with legal issues, such as squatters claiming right of ownership to raw land, or an individual claiming ownership of a house or estate once belonging to an ancestor (often seized or lost in WWII redrawing of borders).

As well, rental scams aimed at foreigners are an ongoing problem. They include the classic "bait-and-switch" and "owners" requesting wired, up-front funds for properties copied and pasted from other ads.

Real Estate Purchasing Essentials: Buying property abroad is obviously a much trickier proposition than doing so at home. The major hurdles include finding a reputable agent and/or developer and legal representative to provide recourse should something go awry.

To get you started, here are some helpful websites addressing real estate fraud and offering sound advice:

Expatica.com's "Top Five Tips for Buying Overseas Property" at Expatica.com/nl/housing/renting/Top-five-tips-for-buying-overseas-property-_18608.html.

US News' "How to Screen an Overseas Developer" at Money.USNews.com/money/blogs/on-retirement/2014/02/03/how-to-screen-an-overseas-developer.

The Law Firm of Arnold & Porter, LLP offers international transactional services and counsel, as well as tips for purchasing abroad at ArnoldPorter.com/publications.cfm?action=advisory&u=TheThreeTsOfPurchasingReal EstateAbroad&id=816.

HEALTHCARE

While the cost of health insurance abroad is typically one's primary focus, the most affordable and comprehensive plan means nothing without a solid healthcare infrastructure offering quality services. With Malaysia, France, Panama, and Uruguay consistently topping the lists of countries with high healthcare standards, more in-depth information for advice and quotes can be found at:

International Living: "The Best Places to Retire Overseas for Affordable and Efficient Health Care": InternationalLiving.com/2014/01/best-places-retire -overseas -affordable-efficient-health-care

AARP: AARP.org/home-garden/livable-communities/best _places_to_retire_abroad

The Association of American Residents Overseas: AARO.org/medical-insurance

Blue Cross Blue Shield Travel/International Health Insurance: GeoBlueTravelInsurance.com/product_overview.cfm **(855) 481-6647**

Cigna Global Health Options: CignaGlobal.com/international-medical-insurance **(877) 539-6295**

UnitedHealth Group Global Health:
   UnitedHealthGroup.com/global, **(800) 328-5979**

HTH Worldwide – Healthcare Technologies for the World
   Traveler: HTHWorldwide.net, **(888) 243-2358**

Medibroker International Health Insurance Specialists:
   Medibroker.com

Allianz Worldwide Care: AllianzWorldwideCare.com

CRIME AND VIOLENCE

Most people are concerned about the level of security in many of the popular expat retirement locations. Take Mexico for instance: While millions of people annually visit from the United States without incident, there are increasing reports of violence in areas once seen as safe, so following local news and bulletin boards for expats is important in checking out a potential foreign location for retirement.

TRY IT ON FOR SIZE . . .

Instead of selling the family home and buying that charming, Italian seaside villa, consider renting out your home and leasing a quaint little flat for a bit while trying your new environment on for size.

Similarly, ongoing political and economic instability in other popular retirement areas such as Ecuador, Argentina, and Thailand could easily change their level of attractiveness for relocation.

To address concerns regarding crime and violence abroad, check with the US State Department for advisories and warnings at:

Travel.State.gov/content/passports/english/alertswarnings.html.
   A similar check for advisories posted for foreigners/travelers from other countries would be worth the time as well.

For Canadian citizens: Travel.GC.ca/travelling/advisories

For citizens of the United Kingdom: Gov.uk/foreign-travel-advice

For citizens of all EU member countries:
   EC.Europa.eu/consularprotection/showMap?tab=4

The following website offers crime statistics by country: Nationmaster.com/country-info/stats/Crime/Total-crimes. For your specific city/town of interest, it's best to search the Internet for relevant articles, expat forums, and blogs.

If you've decided that life abroad is for you, be sure to visit your target relocation destination at least once or twice to get a taste for the lifestyle and to investigate housing. Scams are plenty, and the best way to avoid them is to go to the source. Additionally, exhaustively read articles, blogs, and forums dedicated to your target city. Chat online with American expats living in your new, future hometown, or plan, upon visiting, to join an American expat group meet-up in a safe, public environment in order to make some initial (and potentially quality) contacts there.

When planning to move abroad, be sure to employ a common sense approach to decision-making, always listen to your instincts, and, as much as possible, leave nothing to chance.

These basic "do's and don'ts" should get you on the road to deciding where to settle in retirement:

DaVINCI DO'S

- If funds are tight with respect to living arrangements, consider pooling resources with family members. Fill that empty in-law suite or spare bedroom, or use the extra income to finance an addition.

- If possible, utilize the services of an SRES (Senior Real Estate Specialist) certified agent. They are expressly trained to cater to the needs of those 50 and over in the areas of buying, selling, finance/refinance options, and relocation.

- Avoid any "agent" pressuring you to sign a contract to sell your home to an eager buyer. Legitimate, professional real estate agents don't knock on doors or cold call.

DaVINCI DON'TS

- Don't feel compelled to do business with the first real estate agent you interview, no matter how hard their sales pitch. Do your homework beforehand, ask for references, and hold your ground — you'll know when you've found the agent that's a good fit for you.

- Don't plan on selling the family home and relocating before you've at least visited the target location, or better yet, spent some time there to get a feel for the lifestyle.

- Don't ever invest abroad without securing a reputable agent and legal counsel beforehand.

5

Inheritance

IF YOU ARE LUCKY enough to inherit money or real property from a parent or grandparent, you may still be unlucky enough to get hit with federal and state taxes. Aside from quarrels with other family members about who inherited what and whether it was fair, taxes are the main issue in inheritance.

First, the money or money value of property you inherit was already subject to taxes when it was earned. The person who made you an heir had paid income or capital gains taxes; therefore, a tax on inheritance is double taxation. We must, however, acknowledge that inheritance taxes have a long history, and there are socioeconomic and legal justifications for taxing inheritances, even if we don't like it as taxing the same money twice. This is why groups that oppose inheritance and estate taxes call them "death taxes," as a semantically loaded way to criticize their very existence. On the whole, inheritance and estate taxes fall most heavily on the rich, contributing to the political tone of nearly all the discussion of inheritance taxes.

What's the difference between an estate tax and an inheritance tax? These are legal distinctions that boil down mainly to who is being taxed. An estate tax is imposed on the transfer of the property of a recently deceased individual and paid by the representative of the deceased, usually the executor of the will. The estate tax is a federal tax, independent of heirs.

An inheritance tax is also imposed on the transfer of the property of the deceased, but it is paid by the heirs after the executor has paid estate taxes. The inheritance tax is a state tax and directly targeted to the heirs. We might say that estate and inheritance taxes together represent triple taxation: the deceased already paid income or capital gains taxes; the estate tax is applied, taxing it a second time; and then it is taxed a third time — the inheritance tax.

In the United States, it's important to note that a spouse is almost always considered the natural heir, even against the wishes of the deceased, and that money and property inherited by a spouse is almost always tax-free, with some exceptions for non-citizens and non-residents. But if the heir is a child, a sibling, or a stranger, most states have a sliding scale of taxes for each of those relationships. Historically, inheritance systems favored sons over daughters, and often the eldest son to the exclusion of other sons, but in the United States, starting in colonial times, women (beginning with married women) obtained property rights in their own names and thus the ability to inherit and to leave inheritances. The book *Inheritance and Wealth in America*, an insightful compilation of original essays, traces the history of such tradition and laws, revealing the evolution of present-day practices.

Why Do We Have Inheritance and Estate Taxes?

The rationale for the inheritance tax has two foundations: First, the decedents no longer have property rights, and secondly, society doesn't want to reward people for being born lucky (to wealthy parents). The well-heeled often get the idea that wealth makes them better than the hoi polloi — not subject to the same laws and rules of conduct, and sometimes, entitled to rule. The inheritance tax was designed as a tool to prevent the accumulation of wealth in the hands of a few families.

The inheritance tax is not new, not an American invention, and not in any way related to socialism, as sometimes charged (possibly because the modern estate tax was enacted in the United States in 1916, around the same time as the Russian Revolution in 1917).

Inheritance taxes were imposed as early as Roman times and were widespread during feudal times. The US version of inheritance taxation has a history starting with the political philosophers who influenced the Founding Fathers, starting with John Locke, who said that property ownership is a God-given right, as is the right to bequeath it to heirs, but no one should own excessive amounts of property at the expense of the rest of society. When the rights of one property owner clash with the needs of the rest of society, the state has an obligation to act in the interests of the greater good — the rest of society.

John Locke (1632–1704), Englishman and key figure of the Enlightenment, is important to the history of government because he was among the first to propose the principles on which the United States was founded — that natural law gives all people, equally, the right to life, liberty, and property, independent of a monarch. Government rules only by the consent of the governed. It is the purpose of government to ensure protection of the life, liberty, and property of the governed, and to promote the public good. This is the essence of the "social contract," an intrinsic part of the philosophical underpinnings of the Founding Fathers, who believed the rights and duties of the government and of the governed should be defined in order to create a sustainable society. To these ends, for example, a government should be based on majority rule and the legislative function should be separate from the executive function. A government that fails to do so *should* be overthrown by revolution.

About Locke's views on inheritance, academics quarrel because he wrote that while owning property is a right of natural law, accumulation of wealth should be limited (via taxation) before it became excessive, and that one's wealth should consist of what one had himself earned. But Locke was not the only influential thinker of the day, and others proposed that the good of society trumped accumulation of wealth, and the "good of society" included not permitting rigid class distinctions based on accumulation of wealth. Adam Smith, the original proponent of *laissez-faire* capitalism, objected to inheritance taxes not on any grand principles of natural rights, but pragmatically on the grounds that governments used the proceeds for unproductive purposes, while private hands would use the money for productive ones.

Around the same time, in the late 1700s, a new tenet of law was put forth by English jurist William Blackstone, who said that the right to own property ends with death, and there is no "natural" right to dispose of property after death. Disposing of property after death is a matter of civil law, and to prevent "undue economic disturbances," the state has the right to regulate transfers of property from the dead to the living.

The Founding Fathers were profoundly influenced by these Enlightenment thinkers, and in the end, Blackstone's point of view — that property rights end with death and civil law correctly rules the disposition of the decedent's property — became the core of both the British and American inheritance law and inheritance tax law. Founding Father Thomas Jefferson concurred that property ownership was a natural right, but one that was limited by the needs of the rest of society, and the right ends at death.

The Jeffersonian view has prevailed and been embodied in numerous laws and court cases. The United States has imposed inheritance taxes since the Stamp Tax Act of 1797 (used to finance with the "Undeclared War" with France), repealed in 1802 but re-imposed in 1862, in part to finance the Civil War. Inheritance taxes became a political hot potato in the last years of the 19th century, when utopian and socialist reformers sought to redistribute the tax burden more heavily on the rich. The estate tax became entrenched in the War Act of 1898 (Spanish-American War) and was affirmed in a 1900 Supreme Court case (*Knowlton v. Moore*). Inheritance tax law remains, with multiple changes, to this day, having been written into the 1916 Revenue Act that establishes the income tax.

The inheritance tax got a boost in 1889 from an essay written by industrialist Andrew Carnegie titled "Savage Wealth," also referred to as "The Gospel of Wealth." Carnegie argued that the biggest curse a wealthy man could lay on his children is the burden of extreme wealth, which would deaden their energies and lead them to unproductive lives. Benjamin Franklin wrote much the same way about his son, who was "taking on airs," and warned him not to expect an inheritance. In the end, Franklin bequeathed him some land in Nova Scotia and his books and papers, with the bulk of his estate going to his daughter and other relatives.

Carnegie observed that the heirs to family fortunes often indulged in unhealthy lifestyles and squandered the money. But leaving money to charities was not such a good idea either, because charities tend not to lift the poor out of poverty but only to perpetuate it. He favored philanthropy to new enterprises as a duty of the newly rich to the rest of society that had, in fact, made possible the accumulation of wealth in the first place. "Surplus" wealth could best be put to use by the wealthy themselves, not the state or charities, to alleviate stratification of society into money-based classes. Carnegie himself funded thousands of public libraries and insisted any town getting a Carnegie library had to create a tax to sustain it. Believing the wealth-creator had the best management skills to determine the conditions of philanthropy, Carnegie also supported heavy inheritance taxes.

Carnegie's legacy led to many other do-good foundations established by wealthy families including Ford and Rockefeller, and most recently to The Giving Pledge (GivingPledge.org), organized in 2009 by Microsoft's Bill Gates and investment magnate Warren Buffett to get multimillionaires to donate more than half their fortunes to good causes during either their lifetimes or via will.

Federal Estate Tax

Remember, federal estate taxes are levied against the money and property of the deceased and paid by his or her representative. Estate taxes are paid to the IRS based on the sum of money or the money value left over after the executor pays the debts of the deceased, funeral expenses, and his own fee. You file the tax using IRS Form 706, United States Estate Tax Return. The justification for the tax is that it is a *transfer* of money and property, which is why it's covered as one part of Unified Gift and Estate Tax laws. The IRS puts it this way: "The estate tax is a tax on your *right to transfer property at your death.*" Conversely, the gift tax is one imposed on your right to transfer property during life.

You need to file the form within nine months of your spouse's death and pay the tax on April 15 of the year following your receipt of the inheritance, subject to some tricky exceptions and exemptions. For example, if your spouse passed on January 1, Form

706 is due on or before October 1 (within nine months), even if a surviving spouse applies for a 15-month deferral in order to use the deceased spouse's unused estate tax exemption, called a "portability election." In other words, you have to file the inheritance tax forms with the IRS on time even if no tax payment is due and a status adjustment is going to be made later. Form 706, along with general instructions, can be found at IRS.gov/instructions/i706. For specific questions, call (800) 829-1040.

Portability

The portability election is a new feature that was added to a tax bill in 2010 and made permanent in January 2013 when President Obama signed the American Taxpayer Relief Act, or ATRA. Portability means that the amount of an estate that is exempt from taxation, $5,340,000 as of 2013, can be transferred to the surviving spouse. The exemption will be re-calculated every year for inflation. The top federal estate-tax rate on the largest estates is now 40 percent. Portability means a surviving spouse can get the deceased spouse's unused exemption amount, adding it to his or her own exemption, saving the survivor from having to engage in any special tax-sheltering maneuvers.

Even if the estate you are inheriting falls well below the exclusion exemption at the federal level, you may still want to apply for portability in case your state is among those that taxes inheritances. In some states, the taxing authority looks to the federal filing and in any case, for an estate of any real size, you need to have filed Form 706 to ensure portability for the next generation.

HERE'S HOW IT WORKS

Without portability, consider a couple with $8 million in net worth held in joint title. Spouse A can accept transfer of the entire amount as a right of survivorship with an unlimited marital deduction (if both parties are US citizens). But when Spouse B dies, if the estate is still worth $8 million, after subtracting the $5,340,000 exemption amount, the remaining taxable amount is $2,660,000, and the 40 percent federal inheritance tax is equal to $1,064,000.

With portability, Spouse B's estate can apply the exemption from Spouse A plus the exemption from Spouse B, or a total of

$10,680,000. This is more than the value of the estate, assuming it's still $8 million. There is zero federal inheritance tax due, saving the new heirs $1,064,000 million. But remember, Form 706 has to be filed to get the portability benefit.

State Inheritance Taxes

State inheritance taxes are paid by the heirs of the departed. These laws vary by state and change often, so it's important to check your own state tax laws when considering inheritance taxes. Twenty-one states (and the District of Columbia) apply a state inheritance tax, and the exemptions and other conditions can change from time to time. Ohio repealed the tax effective January 2013 and Indiana's inheritance tax will apply until January 1, 2022. Tennessee's tax will go out of effect on January 1, 2016, and the exemption amount goes up each year until then. Other states are raising the exemption amounts, such as Maine and Rhode Island. Illinois re-instituted the tax in 2011, although the exemption amount was raised to $4 million as of January 1, 2013. Connecticut, in contrast, lowered its exemption from $3.5 million to $2 million.

In 2010, two states eliminated inheritance taxes (Kansas and Oklahoma), and in 2011 North Carolina introduced a tax but repealed it retroactively to January 2013. Hawaii changed the exemption amounts and seems to be the only state that allows portability for spouses. Other states with an estate tax are Washington and Minnesota, each with differing exemptions and conditions. Wills.About.com provides a list and updates, but if you have a real, live inheritance on your hands, you should check your own state government website. You can easily find this information on the Internet by typing in the name of your state and the phrase "inheritance tax."

Tax rates and exemption amounts vary wildly. Rates range from 9.5 percent (Tennessee) to 20 percent (Washington State), and exemption levels vary from $3,500 (Pennsylvania) to $2,750,000 (Vermont). States with estate taxes typically exempt $1 million or less, but the top tax rate tends to be under 20 percent. In New York State, for example, an estate of $5,340,000 would escape federal tax, but $427,200 would be owed in state tax (at a rate of 8 percent). When compared to Florida, which has no state tax, many New Yorkers have decided to move south to reap the financial benefit.

To make life more complicated, some states apply both an estate tax like the federal government and an inheritance tax, to boot. Maryland, for example, imposes an estate tax of up to 16 percent with a $1 million exemption, *plus* a 10 percent inheritance tax on money left to anyone other than the spouse, children, grandchildren, parents, or siblings. A person who wants to leave money to a niece or nephew, friend or business partner should acknowledge they will be subject to an inheritance tax. Note that life insurance policy payouts to an estate are subject to tax as part of the estate, while life insurance policies payable to survivors is not taxable.

The Gift Tax and Exemptions

Philanthropy is promoted by tax exemption of donations to registered charities and other qualified entities. Presumably, the extremely wealthy would follow Carnegie's advice even in the absence of tax exemptions, but there's no doubt that charitable giving is part of tax planning (and ramps up as year-end approaches and the wealthy start figuring how to lower their tax bills).

Even for people without millions to donate to charity, the gift tax exemption is the ideal escape hatch. As described in previous sections,, the federal estate tax and state inheritance taxes can together take as much as 60 percent of an estate (as in the case of Washington state). The remedy — lawful tax avoidance — is to make tax-free gifts before death to reduce the size of the estate. You can make a tax-free gift of up to $14,000 per recipient to as many persons as you wish, with a lifetime tax exemption cap on cumulative gifts totaling $5.34 million (up from $5.25 million in 2013).

The IRS requires that you keep records on gifts because their total will be subtracted from your federal estate tax exemption allotment. As mentioned, your estate, unified with any gifts, is exempt from the tax if it is under $5.34 million. But if you have been making reported gifts *over and above* the annual exempt amounts that total $5.34 million, whatever remains of your estate is subject to the full tax rate of up to 40 percent. In other words, the IRS exempts you from the federal estate tax by either cumulative gifts above the tax-exempt amount or upon probate, but the "lifetime exemption" remains $5.34 million (for 2014).

Really rich people have accountants and lawyers to handle gifts and estate planning, including some fancy footwork when the exclusion amount rose from $5.12 million to $5.25 million in 2012, and now to $5,340,000; however, for most people with an estate under those lofty sums, the gift tax exclusion has two tremendous benefits: Not only does it reduce your taxes in the current tax year, it reduces the uncertainty faced by your heirs.

And if you don't want to face an IRS audit or subject your heirs to one, you need to declare the gifts using Form 709 so that the IRS knows how much of your unified exclusion you have used up. If you made gifts of $1 million over the years above the annual tax-exempt amount, for example, your lifetime unused tax exclusion is now $4.34 million. As long as your gifts are no more than $14,000 per recipient, you do not reduce your lifetime unified gift and estate tax exemption of $5.34 million. In other words, you and your spouse can each give $5.34 million in tax-free gifts during your lifetimes, for a total of $10.68 million before taxation begins.

Married couples share the exclusion during life, a process named "gift-splitting," although the gifts today still reduce the tax exclusion when they both die. This means both the husband and the wife can make a gift to a child of $14,000, tax-free, for a total of $28,000 per year. A popular gift is a contribution to a Section 529 education savings plan, which accumulates and can be withdrawn tax-free when used as intended for college, vocational school, or other accredited institution, and associated expenses. You can even deposit as much as $70,000 at one time ($140,000 for a married couple) and elect that it be considered a five-year gift (meaning you can't make any additional annual gifts to the 529 beneficiary during the five-year period).

Most people don't think about reducing the size of their estates by using tax-free gifts because they have estates under $5.34 million that will escape federal estate taxes, although they may face state inheritance taxes. And yet using gifts to reduce current income taxes and to clarify the inheritance positions of the pool of heirs may be an excellent idea.

Why You Should Think About Inheritance

Even at the level of inherited property of little or no monetary value, it's always a good idea for people to know what to expect and also what they are leading others to expect. This is because heirs will squabble over the smallest things, sometimes ripping families apart. If you want some memento in particular from your parents, you should ask for it, and you should also turn around and ask your heirs which things of yours they would like to have to remember you by.

This is the universal advice of family counselors and estate lawyers, who say that bringing inheritance details out in the open is the only way to avoid heartbreak later. Of course, a person who tries to dominate and control putative heirs with threats of writing them out of the will don't like this advice. Before you dismiss a fight over inheritance as never possible in your family, consider that just about every family ends up with someone having hurt feelings at the least and a titanic court battle at the worst. In *Blood & Money: Why Families Fight Over Inheritance and What To Do About*, P. Mark Accettura reveals what's behind this set of psychological conflicts that are not well understood even today, ranging from relatively benign sibling rivalry ("Mother always loved you best!") to the utterly antagonistic, such as a person leaving a "toxic" will to stir up trouble where none existed before.

An important point is that the thought of inheritance, whether giving or receiving, raises unwelcome thoughts of death, and the United States is a society that likes to sweep death under the rug. Heirs may not be petty or greedy — they may just be uncomfortable when it comes to broaching the subject. Those of certain faiths find comfort in the idea of an afterlife, and the secular fend off the idea of death with glib talk of bucket lists, but mostly we avoid talk of death and shield children from death. What happens after death is man's number one question; the idea that there may be nothing — the existential black hole — is truly terrifying. No wonder we think it would be graceless to speak of Dad's watch when we can barely bring ourselves to think of Dad dying, much less talk with Dad about it. It would be foolish to imagine that everyone involved is going to behave rationally and appropriately about inheritance when they can't bear to think about death itself.

One thing we get almost no warning about is the potential for crooked family insiders, suspiciously friendly strangers, or estate lawyers poised to "hijack" an inheritance. The sums can be staggering. One estimate is that IRA savings of the baby boomer generation are $25 trillion and the total value of baby boomer estates changing hands over the next twenty years is $100 trillion. Inheritance theft stays under the radar of law enforcement and hardly ever makes the evening news for many reasons — people are unwilling to admit they were bamboozled or they may not even know that a theft has occurred because only part of an estate was taken. A relatively typical case is where a person leaves bequests to a slew of nieces and nephews, and the bulk of an estate to an only son. The son, as the primary heir, simply tears up the will naming the nieces and nephews. If the nieces and nephews were never apprised of their inheritance and had no evidence the will even existed, there is no one to make a case that a crime has even occurred, and the son effectively makes off with the inheritances of his cousins.

The targets of inheritance-hijacking come in two forms: the person who has no spouse or close family members, and those who are in declining physical and mental health and therefore vulnerable to outside influences (often caregivers). A particularly vulnerable subset is elderly folks who marry much younger people — marrying is the easiest way of swindling a late spouse's survivors out of their inheritance. Another group is those who are simply not willing to make any estate plan at all, setting off a free-for-all.

The hijackers consist of both family and non-family parties. In family situations, it can be a family member who is unscrupulous and clever, like the son having the same name as his father who signs his father's home title and other ownership papers and forgets to put in the "Jr." Technically this is fraud, but it is hardly ever prosecuted. Non-family theft comes in the form of caregivers, second spouses, church or club friends, neighbors, friendly strangers, and dishonest estate lawyers. If you are planning to give or receive an inheritance, you can take a self-assessment test on whether you are susceptible to inheritance hijacking at RCAdamski.com/design/pdfs/Risk-to-your-inheritance-quiz.pdf.

Inheritance can be a touchy business. Utilize the following "dos and don'ts" in order to avoid some common pitfalls:

DaVINCI DO'S

- Inheritance tax is paid by your heirs, so learn the laws of your state, as each state varies and laws change often.

- Although broaching the subject may be a bit uncomfortable, talk about inheritance with those from whom you expect to inherit and those who expect to inherit from you. If you want a memento, ask for it; as well, you should ask your heirs if there is anything in particular they would like. Write it down and incorporate those notes into the will.

- Make tax-free gifts — the IRS allows up to $14,000 per recipient per year to as many persons as you wish, with a lifetime tax exemption cap on cumulative gifts totaling $5.34 million.

DaVINCI DON'TS

- Don't be remiss in applying for portability (the remaining estate tax exemption of your deceased spouse) if your state is among those that taxes inheritances. IRS form 706 must be filed within nine months of your spouse's death.

- Don't forget to keep records of gifts. The IRS requires this because their total will be subtracted from your federal estate tax exemption allotment.

- Don't let your estate fall prey to hijackers. Contact a reputable real estate attorney to safeguard your inheritors or if you feel your inheritance has been hijacked. A Better Business Bureau Certified real estate attorney can be found at BBB.com.

6

Wills and Trusts

NO ONE IS IMMORTAL. Everybody dies. We all know that, and yet a very large percentage of people (over half) choose not to draw up a will — even a hand-written, makeshift version. Dying without a will is referred to as dying "intestate," and invites the state government to poke its nose into your business. In fact, a will is a person's instructions to the government — a judge — on how to distribute his property. You may think it's the choice of the person's family, but that is true only in cases where there is very little property involved. In most other cases, and especially when there is a lot of property, the state gets to decide on behalf of the survivors and the estate.

We have all heard horror stories of people dying intestate and the courts taking decades to distribute the property. Jimi Hendrix' estate took thirty years to settle. Pablo Picasso's estate took six years and cost $30 million. The most famous person to die intestate was Abraham Lincoln, and he was a lawyer.

Why Do People Fail to Prepare for the Inevitable?

Avoiding writing a will doesn't keep your heirs out of the legal system — it just makes it harder for them. Wanting to avoid the legal system is understandable; we all know (or think we know) it's expensive, time-consuming, and often doesn't deliver justice due to legal trickery on the part of corrupt attorneys. A famous story details our disdain for lawyers: Marilyn Monroe's estate took in $1.6 million from movie royalties from her death in 1960 to 1980. Her heirs got $101,229, her creditors got $372,136 and the lawyers got over $1 million. That's why we hate lawyers.

Survey research from Pew finds that lawyers are the most despised professional in the United States, followed by corporate business executives and journalists. In all three instances, the professional is seen as heartless and out for himself at any cost. We revere the rule of law (over the whims of men) as a foundation of democracy, but we abhor lawyers.

Get over it... and beat them at them at their own game. One of the revolutionary advances of the baby boomer generation is to fight back against "authority," in this case the legal profession, by educating themselves. A good way is to use do-it-yourself legal forms in order to become familiar with the requirements, process, and jargon of will-writing.

Dying Without a Will

If you die intestate (without a will), the state will determine who gets your property — almost always your spouse and children, or other closest relatives, starting with your brother or sister. If you do not have relatives that can be found, your property goes to the state. If you have minor children and no spouse, the probate judge will decide who gets the responsibility of caring for them.

Right away you can see how probate issues can become horribly tangled. Probate is the term describing the legal process of transferring property from the "estate" of the deceased to the parties named in the will, and it starts with determining whether the will is valid. The probate process is a checklist of items that have to qualify under the law and satisfy the probate court judge. Debts and taxes have to be paid before the heirs get their inheritance, so, for example, if your brother lent you $100,000, and the liquid assets in the estate are worth less than $100,000, your brother could conceivably ask the court to force your spouse to sell the house to get the money to repay the debt. Of course, your brother would have to prove to the court that the debt existed in a correctly documented manner.

Probate laws are state laws, not federal laws, and as a general rule, your property will be probated in the state in which you resided. Your stock portfolio may technically be located in the city where your broker is headquartered, but for probate purposes, it is considered to be located in the state where you lived. Real estate is an exception. If you live in New York State but own a cabin in Maine, the cabin has to be probated in Maine. Let's say you left the cabin in Maine to someone not related to you, or to someone "less related" than your daughter or son, like a cousin's child. The daughter or son may have the right to contest the will in Maine under Maine probate law.

Lines of succession — who inherits and in what order — vary from state to state, although many states have adopted something named the Uniform Probate Code (UPC), whose purpose is to simplify and standardize the processes and rules of distributing the property. One aspect of the Uniform Probate Code is protection of spouses and children, who are entitled to some minimum amount of the property even if the writer of the will tries to cut them out entirely. Think of a case where a man has divorced his first wife with whom he has children, and remarried. He wants to leave everything to the second wife and children and nothing to the first wife and children. In most instances, this would not be allowed. Or a person has adopted another adult and wants to leave everything to this adopted person and nothing to his real biological children. Such a will would be contestable under the UPC.

The UPC was adopted in full by 16 states, and many of the other 34 states have adopted some aspects of it. Note that in all things legal, Louisiana is an exception, with its laws based on the Napoleonic Code. The 16 states are Alaska, Arizona, Colorado, Florida, Hawaii, Idaho, Maine, Michigan, Minnesota, Montana, Nebraska, New Mexico, North Dakota, South Carolina, South Dakota, and Utah. If your will is going to be probated in a state that has not adopted the UPC, you can look up specific provisions by Googling "probate" and the name of your state. That will take you to the probate court website (as well as providing numerous ads for probate lawyers and the occasional interesting article). You probably don't want to read the UPC document itself — it's impenetrable — but the most recently revised (February 2013) edition is available on-line. The document can be accessed at UniformLaws.org/shared/docs/probate%20code/upc%202010.pdf.

The line of succession — the hierarchy of heirs — can get very confusing. For one thing, it uses words that we don't typically use in the course of ordinary life, like "consanguinity" and "escheat." Every state has its own default succession rules. Here is one version of the order of preference for inheritance, but be aware that this list will not hold in every state:

1. Surviving spouse

2. Children

3. Parents

4. Brothers and sisters and their lineal descendants

5. Grandparents and their lineal descendants

6. Next of kin

7. If no next of kin, then escheat (default) to the state

In some states, the surviving spouse gets the entire estate, even if estranged; in others, the spouse must share the estate with surviving parents. Be sure to check whether your state has "parental inheritance." Spouses do not get everything when there are children, too — usually one-third to one-half, with the remainder going to the children. In some states, the spouse gets one-half of the estate even if the deceased has children from a previous marriage.

States also vary by how far they will go in searching the line of succession to find an heir before deciding the estate belongs to the state. In New York State, for example, the line goes as far as to the great grand-children, but in other states it could go as far as first cousins three times removed (the great grandchildren of your first cousin). Once the line of succession is exhausted and no heirs are found, the estate escheats, or defaults, to the state.

Every state has rules defining how small an estate has to be to avoid probate. The amounts vary all over the place, from $50,000 in Arizona (personal property like a checking account and jewelry, not including real estate, which is called "real property") to $200,000 in Wyoming. You can get a state-by-state shortcut listing at the always useful Nolo.com (Nolo.com/legal-encyclopedia/ probate-shortcuts-in-your-state-31020.html). When the amount of property is small enough to qualify for unsupervised adminis- tration, the representative (usually the spouse or family member) submits a simple declaration to the court. If the estate is uncon- tested, that's it — probate is avoided. In practice, in the absence of anyone contesting the distribution of property, states do not chase down an heir who doesn't submit the declaration to the court.

The Essence of a Will

The essence of a will is defining what you want to happen to your money, property, minor children, and pets when you die. If you fail to define your wishes with absolute clarity and in terms that would be impossible to misinterpret, anyone wanting to contest the will may get enough of a foothold to legally challenge it. It seems obvi- ous that if you don't like a blood relative and that person would be next in line to inherit from you, you should take some action to get your way — not what cultural history or the law might dictate. A will also allows you to name the person who is going to carry out your wishes — the executor, or representative to the court. If you neglect to name an executor, in most cases the state takes over that function by appointing a lawyer to do the job, to be paid out of the estate (with outcomes you possibly wouldn't have approved of).

Writing a Will

The conditions of a valid will are few but fixed — they must be met for the will to be valid.

   1. You must be of sound mind. Unless you are confined to a mental-health facility or someone contests your will on the grounds you were of unsound mind, the state is willing to believe that you were "of sound mind." While soundness of mind is the default assumption, extreme old age (90 to 100+) is sometimes used to challenge wills, on the grounds that anyone that old must be mentally incompetent to some degree.

   If there is any question as to one's mental state at the time the will was executed, a letter from a medical professional is useful. The crux of the much publicized case of Mrs. Brooke Astor was whether she was mentally competent to have signed changes to her 2002 will in 2003 and 2004. She was 100 years of age in 2002, but falling prey to dementia, and the changes to the will were deemed inconsistent with the intent of the original will. The court determined she had been tricked by her son into signing later versions while of unsound mind. The trial jurors convicted the son, who was himself 85 at the time, on 14 criminal counts, including fraud, and Mrs. Astor's estate lawyer was convicted, as well, of conspiracy, scheming to defraud, and forgery. In the end, the state attorney general used a combination of wills, including one from 1997, to settle Mrs. Astor's estate.

Judges rarely want to declare someone mentally incompetent, but someone challenging the document may prevail by demonstrating with a "preponderance of the evidence" that the person lacked the mental capacity to sign a valid will. Preponderance means that the case for unsoundness is greater than the case for soundness, and both sides usually present witnesses, medical records, and doctors' testimony. In the Astor case, it was the grandson challenging the last version of the will and bringing forth witnesses, including long-time friends and medical professionals, to prove that Mrs. Astor's mental capacity had deteriorated significantly by the time of the signing of the 2003 and 2004 versions.

How do you prove you are of sound mind, and thus qualified to sign your will, especially if you are eccentric or sometimes forgetful? The key is that you know what the will means — that its purpose is to distribute your property after death. You also must know the property that is at stake and the names and relationships of the heirs. You will is valid though you may have wild opinions and prejudices, you are illiterate, or you are so physically feeble you can barely write your name. The will of an alcoholic or drug addict is valid as long as he was not under the influence at the time of signing. These are drawbacks to, but not signs of "testamentary incapacity."

2. You have to sign and date the will in the presence of two witnesses, who then put their own signatures and date. Some states require three witnesses. The witnesses don't have to read the will, but in most states cannot be heir to anything in the will. Wills do not have to be notarized, but it's not a bad idea to do the multiple signings in the presence of a notary and pay the nominal fee to get the notary stamp and seal it if you expect a challenge, or if the local probate court is particularly persnickety. It can't harm and might help.

What about a "holographic" will? This is a will written entirely in the person's handwriting and signed and dated. Twenty-six states recognize holographic wills as valid, with most states not requiring a witness, and sometimes not even requiring the date. Despite the fact that roughly half of the states find such a document valid, it is always better to err on the side of caution by hiring a professional to handle the legalities, especially when assets and heirs are numerous.

Though it is recommended that one seeks counsel when executing any legal document, you do not necessarily need a lawyer to write your will. With cases involving a complicated family situation or property you want to distribute unconventionally, however, it is always best to consult a lawyer.

Online will forms, which are recommended only as a starting point, can be found free at LawDepot.com, and TotalLegal.com. Although there is no shortage of places to get a free form, you might like Nolo.com, which charges $34.99 for the form but also contains many pages of useful information. LegalZoom.com (which advertises on TV) charges $69 for the basic version and $79 for the comprehensive version, and claims to offer all kinds of extras like archival quality paper. The Quicken WillMaker Plus was designed by Nolo, and comes with extras like a power of attorney form. It costs $42.99, but can be found for less on eBay, in office-supply stores, and elsewhere. Again, these online forms are best used as your own, initial resource, which will later be drafted into a legally binding document by a professional.

Changing and Revoking Your Will

No sooner have you completed your will than your favorite granddaughter admires a painting on your wall and you decide you would like to bequeath it to her. This means you have to add an amendment, referred to as a "codicil," to your will. The problem is that you have to go through signing in front of two (or three) witnesses all over again, and inherent in the codicil process, of course, is that you are still of sound mind and not been subject to undue influence.

If you elect have an entirely new will drafted, you must have the previous document revoked, or "repudiated," which is done by literally shredding or burning it. Don't leave it lying around for heirs to squabble over. Multiple wills are the stuff of Agatha Christie whodunits, not modern life.

"Undue influence" is a factor increasingly at the forefront of disputes over wills as a form of elder abuse, as in the Brooke Astor case. Undue influence is carried out by a person in a position of power over another, like a caregiver or care-giving relative. The influence can range from manipulative flattery to any other form of persuasion that overwhelms the free will of the will-writer. Undue influence is less harsh than duress, which includes blackmail and the threat of force or use of force.

Undue influence is tricky. One element is that the will-maker has to be proven to have been susceptible or vulnerable to persuasion, which is walking a fine-line with respect to the mental-soundness criterion. A person who is psychologically or physically dependent on another might be considered susceptible to undue influence. The second factor is opportunity, and that typically arises in the form of a confidential relationship. Obviously a confidential relationship exists between husband and wife, parent and child, etc., so the opportunity factor is most suspicious when the undue influence is exercised by a guardian, doctor, pastor, or other non-family party.

Someone who is accused of exercising undue influence has to be shown to have an inclination to do so, by keeping other people away, by discouraging outside advice, and other means. Finally, undue influence has to take a concrete form, such as a massive and abrupt change in the will strictly for the self-benefit of the accused party. Legal-Dictionary.TheFreeDictionary.com has this to say about undue influence:

> Nevertheless, courts will examine the facts closely before finding that a transaction has been tainted by undue influence. Mere suspicion, surmise, or conjecture of overreaching is insufficient. The law permits loved ones and confidants to advise and comfort those in need of their support without fear of litigation. Courts are also aware that the doctrine of undue influence can be used as a sword by the vindictive and avaricious who seek to invalidate a perfectly legal transaction for personal gain. When undue

influence is found to have altered a transaction, however, courts will make every effort to return the parties to the same position they would have occupied had the over-reaching not occurred.

The Center for Elders and the Courts (EldersAndCourts.org, 757-259-1593) publishes material showing that undue influence is on the rise against elders, and court personnel are advised to be on the lookout as the last public bastion against such abuse, even if the older person is not making a complaint. The key issues are capacity and consent. Capacity is a set of mental skills, such as memory and logic, which everyone uses every day. But it can be hard to determine capacity in older persons and may take professionals to evaluate. Consent is the ability to understand the transaction at hand and have the judgment to choose or reject it. In the absence of capacity and consent, undue influence can easily ensue, exploiting trust and dependence to gain control over the elder person's decision-making or assets.

How do you know if someone is trying to put undue influence on you? Every case is different, but one good clue is if the influencer wants to be present when the will is drawn up, excluding others, or when the influencer offers to bring a lawyer over for a home visit to prepare the will.

Contesting a Will

Courts rarely declare a will to be invalid, but challenging a will can get a court to change some of the provisions. The law does not allow anyone, other than a presumed heir (in the case of an intestate death) or a named beneficiary of a will, to challenge a will. This keeps strangers from claiming to be long-lost relatives. The only way a person can challenge a will after not being presumed an heir or named is to charge "tortuous interference," meaning the testator was influenced to reduce or eliminate the inheritance.

The four reasons to contest a will are:

1. The will was not signed according to state law.
2. The testator lacked the mental capacity to sign a will.
3. The testator was unduly influenced.
4. The will was fraudulently procured.

Two other situations arise that don't fall under these four rules. The first is "dead-hand control," in which the beneficiary has to meet certain conditions, such as to marry into a particular faith to get the inheritance. Believe it or not, unless a dead-hand-control clause is contrary to public policy (such as being illegal), the court will usually enforce it.

The second situation is the no-contest clause, also called the penalty clause. This is a provision in the will that says if a beneficiary challenges the will, he will be deprived of the inheritance. Obviously, only someone specifically named in the will or in the state's natural succession has an incentive to challenge a will with a no-contest clause. Weirdly, if the will is deemed invalid for any of the four reasons, the penalty clause is invalid, too, so that an intestate heir can end up inheriting in the end. Challenging a will is a lengthy and expensive process — one to be embarked upon only when the stakes are worth it and the evidence is substantial. Even so, challengers sometimes succeed in getting an out-of-court settlement from the estate manager just to make them go away.

One of the most famous cases involving a challenge to a will was Leona Helmsley, the owner of a hotel empire who had cheated on her taxes and spent eighteen months in prison for it. She was nicknamed "the queen of mean" in the New York tabloid press. Her will cut out two grandchildren, but left $12 million to her Maltese dog. The disinherited grandchildren successfully challenged the will on the grounds that Mrs. Helmsley must have been of unsound mind to leave $12 million to a dog. They got $6 million each, and the probate judge was also persuaded to cut the dog's trust fund to $2 million. The executors managed the hotel empire and the investment portfolio, earning $4.5 million in the first year (of the five years it took for the will to be probated in full), or $900,000 for each of the five executors. This is still under the New York state cap on executor compensation of two percent of the estate, which would have been $200 million. Meanwhile, the state's representative, the attorney general, complained the lengthy and expensive process was depriving the ultimate beneficiaries and charities of the proceeds of the estate.

In summary: Don't give the state the right to distribute your property or appoint a guardian for your children after you die. Write a will! If you are in a state that allows a handwritten (holographic) will, take an hour and do it. Or get a free or inexpensive form online and fill it out. Unless you have a lot of property or a complicated family situation, preparing you own will is easy and fast. Deprive those probate lawyers of the chunk of your money that they will get if the court has to appoint one of them because you died without a will.

Do You Need a Living Trust, Too?

A will tells the state how you want your money and property distributed after you die. In many instances, and inevitably when the amounts are large or the will is complicated or contested, the probate process takes many months — often a year or more. In contrast, a living trust allows you to get a head-start on distribution *before* you die. Upon your death, money and property in the trust goes immediately to the heirs, bypassing the probate process and avoiding court and attorney fees.

A revocable living trust can take the place of a will if it is comprehensive enough, although it is not advisable to go without a will and to rely on the trust alone. There are some assets, like your checking account and your car that you wouldn't want to place in a trust. If you have minor children, in most states, a will is the better document to name a guardian. If you are going to become the beneficiary of someone else's will or trust, you can't transfer title to property to your own trust that you do not yet own. And if you want to disinherit someone who is in the natural line of succession, a will is the appropriate instrument. If you are forming a living trust, on the whole you should have a will, too. The Nolo book by Denis Clifford, *Make Your Own Living Trust*, recommends a "backup will" (and provides the forms).

WHAT IS A REVOCABLE LIVING TRUST?

The kind of trust we are talking about here is the "revocable living trust," although you might want to be aware that other types of trusts can be designed for different purposes and situations. These include credit shelter trusts (CST), incentive trusts, generation-skipping trusts, charitable reminder trusts, and irrevocable life insurance trusts. (See the following sections.)

When you create a trust, you transfer ownership of your property to a trustee to hold on behalf of someone else, usually children or grand-children but also organizations of varying purpose.

A trust can be formed as a living trust, while you are still alive, or after death as part of your will. A living trust does not require a separate tax identification number and transactions between the individual and the trust are recorded for tax purposes on the individual tax records and return. In contrast, a trust that is set up after a person's death becomes a new legal entity that requires its own tax ID — you cannot use the decedent's Social Security number. A tax identification number can be obtained online from the IRS website (Form SS-4). Technically, the tax ID is a federal Employer Identification Number (EIN).

While you are alive, you can buy, sell, and transfer assets in the trust, or direct a trustee to do the job, just as though you still owned title to the assets. You, as the "grantor," can name yourself as the trustee, and most people do. You still effectively control the assets. The beneficiary has no right to any of the money or assets in the trust while you are still alive. An additional trustee can be an individual or a firm, or there can be several trustees, each with a defined role. A trust performs the function of separating the title or ownership of the property from the party that gets the benefits of the property, including (usually) eventual, full ownership. A trustee is literally given title to the trust property, but is charged, contractually, to act for the good of the beneficiary. This is known as "fiduciary duty."

Somewhat confusingly, you can be the grantor (also called a settler), a trustee, *and* a beneficiary of the trust all at once, as long as there is one other trustee or one other beneficiary. If you fail to name a second trustee to whom legal title can be transferred, a court will appoint one on behalf of the beneficiary. This pretty much defeats the purpose of a living trust, which is to keep the state out of your business.

A living trust allows you to arrange (and rearrange) your affairs long in advance of your death. You can perform this function yourself or leave it to a trustee. Arranging your affairs ahead of time sounds like a really good idea, but if you are leaving management to the trustee, be perfectly certain that you've chosen the right person for the job. It may seem too obvious to mention, but the whole idea in appointing a particular individual as a trustee is that you actually trust that person. Unfortunately, abuse of trust is all too common, and even worse, the dishonest fiduciary is often a family member — and a close one. If you Google "breach of fiduciary trust," you will get well over two million hits. A lot of them are ads for lawyers, of course, but there is also a vast amount of literature based on both obscure and celebrity cases, as well as special circumstances (most recently, pertaining to hedge funds, which are not relevant to our purposes).

A person harmed by a breach of fiduciary duty can sue for recovery of lost or stolen money and property, but if the money and property was truly lost, he will be out of luck. (At least a convicted fiduciary cannot escape paying damages by declaring bankruptcy.) It is therefore essential that, before you begin, you either know someone who will be 100 percent trustworthy, or resign yourself to hiring a lawyer, who may become the trustee himself or assign the job to another or to a bank or trust company.

ADVANTAGES OF A LIVING TRUST

The primary purpose of a living trust is to avoid probate, not to avoid taxes. The estate and inheritance taxes described in Chapter 5 are not affected by the formation of a living trust (except a special form named an AB trust, which keeps the deceased person's estate separate from that of the surviving spouse). In other words, a living trust is not a tax deferral or tax reduction strategy. But if you own real estate in multiple states, a living trust is its own "paperwork-reduction act," because you are avoiding probate in more than one state.

In addition to avoiding probate, a living trust keeps the courts out of your business by having the trustee manage your affairs if you are suddenly incapacitated. In the absence of a trust, if you have a stroke or otherwise become incapable of managing your affairs, the court may appoint a guardian or conservator — someone not of your choosing. When you form a living trust, you name your own trustee ahead of time.

Another benefit of a living trust is that, if your beneficiaries are minor children or adult children who are financially inept, the trust can be written in such a way as to defer control of the assets until specific ages or to dole out benefits in a manner you deem prudent. Another virtue of a living trust is that they are very, very hard to contest. When a will is contested, the deceased can be deemed as having been incompetent or under duress on the day the will was signed. But to invalidate a living trust, someone contesting the trust would have to demonstrate it was invalid on every day of its existence. In fact, you can specify in your trust that anyone who contests the trust is disinherited by the very fact of the challenge, the same no-contest clause mentioned in the section on wills. If you have quarrelsome heirs, this is probably a very good idea.

As a general rule, assets in the trust are not frozen when a trust is contested, as occurs when a will is contested, so that even if a litigious party challenges the trust, your heirs will get what you wanted them to get. Unless the state freezes a bank account until inheritance taxes are paid, for example, the beneficiary can claim the money in a bank account by simply presenting the death certificate and personal identification.

A revocable living trust means is it changeable while you are still alive. You can revoke any or all provisions and re-arrange them. You can re-write a will, too, but as noted in the section on wills, it may be contested on the grounds that you were not of sound mind when the last will was made, and by then, you are not around any longer to defend yourself. Finally, a trust is a private arrangement and so is the transfer of property to your heirs under the terms of the trust, unlike the probate process, which may expose details of your estate to the public.

DISADVANTAGES OF A LIVING TRUST

You have to be willing to maintain good records or pay someone else to do it. That includes setting up the trust in the first place, which entails transferring titles to the trust, and continually updating assets added or subtracted from the trust. There may be fees payable to the state associated with changing title and there will be fees payable to the trustee if he is doing the administrative work. The administrative work can be onerous if there is a lot of property, complex properties, or complicated properties (like Subchapter S companies, real estate in foreign countries, and other issues). Law firms, banks, and trust companies charge varying fees to maintain these records.

A living trust does not exempt you from federal estate and gift taxes, but as noted in Chapter 5, these taxes are not due until after your death, and in any case, the large majority of estates escape these taxes because the hurdle is so high — $5.34 million for estates and gift taxes cumulatively over your life. You can give anyone up to $14,000 per year per person without incurring the gift tax for a lifetime tax-free maximum of $5.34 million, or $14,000 to nineteen persons every year for twenty years. You can give unlimited gifts without tax (or eating into your cumulative lifetime gift-tax amount) to a spouse who is a US citizen, to tax-exempt charitable organizations, and to pay medical bills and school tuition.

Forming a living trust does not protect your assets from creditors, lawsuits, or divorce since it is the nature of a revocable trust that you can take assets out of it, which a creditor or divorce court can force you to do. The Nolo website points out that to protect assets, you would need an irrevocable trust:

> Wealthy people who are worried about lawsuits may create very complex trusts, often set up with an offshore trustee. They may also set up limited liability companies or entities called 'family limited partnerships.' If you're concerned about creditors and lawsuits, there are also simpler methods to protect assets, such as putting your money in assets that your state protects from creditors. (For example, even if you file for bankruptcy, you can keep the money in your retirement plan accounts; and in some states creditors can't take your house, no matter how much it's worth.) And of course, you can buy insurance.

SPECIAL TRUST CASES

For purposes of avoiding probate and ensuring your wishes are carried out, the revocable living trust is a good option. If you do not have a substantial estate, you can find an inexpensive way to establish your revocable living trust. The Nolo book, *Make Your Own Living Trust* by Denis Clifford (who also wrote *Plan Your Estate*), contains a wealth of information, as does the website, which contains updates, videos, and blogs. The same companies that offer do-it-yourself wills (such as LegalZoom.com) also offer huge amounts of free information.

If, however, you have a substantial estate, a living trust may be only the first step in a wider estate plan that will encompass more complicated issues, including tax minimization. For that, you will need the assistance of a tax accountant or lawyer, and possibly a different kind of trust. Nolo's Clifford warns that if you want to create the special-case trusts named here, you really do need an estate-planning lawyer.

Generation-Skipping Trust (GST)

Owners of very large estates used to create generation-skipping trusts to avoid estate tax on grandfather's estate, then grandmother's, then each of the parents. The trust would leave the bulk of the estate to the grandchildren, with only the income from the trust given to the children. But in 1976, Congress closed the loophole with a GST tax, which expired for a while, but was recently made permanent, effective January 2, 2013, with the signing of the American Taxpayer Relief Act of 2012. The GST transfer tax is applicable to "related individuals more than one generation away and to unrelated individuals more than 37.5 years younger." (Mondaq.com.) The GST tax is 40 percent on amounts over $5,340,000 in 2014, and assessed against the trust when the middle generation dies. The tax implications of GST can quickly become complicated, especially when you factor in estate taxes and gift taxes.

Credit Shelter Trust (CST)

A credit-shelter trust is designed to hold the assets of an estate equal to the tax-free amount that the decedent didn't use. As noted in Chapter 5 on inheritance, you can transfer $5.34 million — called the "exclusion amount" — to someone, free of federal estate tax. After a person dies, any part of the exclusion amount that is left over, unused, can be applied to fund a credit shelter trust, also called a "bypass trust."

The credit shelter trust is related to the AB trust used by married couples, and embodied in the portability provision of current tax law. As previously discussed, portability means that if one spouse dies without having used up the entire federal estate tax exemption, the remaining exclusion amount is added to the surviving spouse's exclusion amount. Therefore, a married couple can pass on $10.68 million to their heirs using portability, with no need for an AB trust.

Portability doesn't remove the value of an AB trust under special circumstances, though. An AB trust can come in handy when the spouses have previous marriages, and thus different sets of beneficiaries. This can get tricky, as when a second spouse is named trustee for the first spouse's children or a spouse wants to tie down assets (like a house) to specific conditions. AB trusts might be useful when a beneficiary is financially inept or has special needs. Finally, an AB trust may overcome the lack of portability in some states that have not adopted it. For the credit-shelter trust to work in the absence of portability, the couple has to divide up their assets about equally for purposes of putting the assets into the revocable living trust. Leaving assets in a joint account defeats the purpose. This is just one of the many reasons lawyers, and even proponents of do-it-yourself documents, advise that special trusts require an attorney's guidance.

Charitable Remainder Trusts

If you have a great deal of money and assets, forming your own charitable trust allows you to donate tax-free before and after death. Most people don't have a large enough estate to justify forming a charitable trust, and besides, charitable trusts are irrevocable and require that you give up control of the trust property. You can still be the beneficiary of some or all of the income produced by the property, but in order to obtain tax-exempt status from the IRS, you have to distance yourself from the management and the "remainder" of the trust's property has to be independent of you and your heirs. The paperwork involved in forming a charitable remainder trust can be formidable. (See IRS.gov/Charities-&-Non-Profits/Private-Foundations.)

The charitable remainder trust has a double tax advantage: The trust property has already been turned over to the charity, and since it didn't belong to you, is not subject to the estate tax. If you have property that has gone up in value by a large amount since you acquired it, you can avoid capital gains tax by donating the property to the trust. (Colleges and universities, whose alumni funds are technically a form of charitable trust, often mention this point.) And if you donate property that is not income-producing to the charity, it can sell the asset to buy something that is income-producing — for you — without paying capital gains taxes itself.

The more immediate advantage is that you can take an income tax deduction for the donation, spread out over five years. It's not a straight, one-for-one deduction, though. The IRS will deduct the value of the property donated from the amount of income from the property you will get back from the charity. How on earth does it do that? The IRS has a formula involving your life expectancy, interest rates, and the terms of the trust. Let's say you donate $100,000 and expect to get $25,000 back in income from the charity over the five years. The value of your gift, and therefore your income tax deduction, is now $75,000.

In most instances, income you receive from a charitable remainder trust comes in the form of a fixed annuity (which relieves the charity of matching a specific percentage return), or a percentage of the total value of the assets, reassessed every year. The latter is better than receiving an annuity because it accounts for inflation. Note that the IRS requires you to take at least 5 percent of the value of the trust every year.

Private Foundations

Foundations are tax-exempt, non-profit organizations started by you or your family with a substantial, initial gift. Charitable contributions are distributed as grants to public charities and other private foundations. Fidelity is perhaps the biggest name in private foundation programs, carrying on the American philanthropic tradition. A description and list of "key characteristics" of private foundations are provided by Fidelity Charitable at FidelityCharitable.org/giving-strategies/give/foundations.shtml, (800) 262-6935. Some of these features include a potential 30 percent immediate tax deduction on cash gifts, full control over granting, and full control over investment management.

The Council on Foundations offers practical, helpful, and easy-to-understand information on starting a foundation, at COF.org, **(800) 673-9036**.

Some other reputable institutions/companies include:

Bank of America at BankOfAmerica.com/philanthropic/privatefoundations.go, **(877) 898-7323**.

Schwab Charitable at SchwabCharitable.org/, (800) 746-6216.

PNC Foundation at www1.pnc.com/pncfoundation/
charitable_trusts.html, **(888) 762-6111**.

Whittier Trust Company at WhittierTrust.com/
philanthropic.html, **(626) 441-5111**.

Fiduciary Duty

Whether you have a simple revocable trust or a fancy version, including a charitable remainder trust, you need at least one trustee. Choosing a trustee can be as important a life decision as choosing a spouse or a doctor. Should it be a person you already know (and will that person outlive you)? If you choose an institution like a bank, you may get a series of inexperienced juniors (unless you are rich enough to fit into the high-net-worth or wealth management department), and you will almost certainly pay more for institutional oversight than individual management. And don't allow someone to remain trustee who is no longer a reliable and trusted member of your circle, like keeping your ex-brother-in-law as trustee long after he divorced your sister and ran off to Bora Bora.

The concept of trusts and fiduciary duty arose out of the first trusts in England during the time of the Crusades (when the trustees refused to return landed estates to returning crusaders until the king and his government finally decided in favor of the returning crusaders). We have, therefore, had many centuries for trust law to be debated, defined, and refined, and vast case law to accumulate. In the United States, the Uniform Trust Code provides a model. Like the Uniform Probate Code described earlier, it was adopted in full by some states, borrowed from in other states, and ignored entirely in yet a third set of states (and Louisiana stands alone). The American College of Trust and Estate Counsel (ACTEC.org, (202) 684-8460) provides a list of the twenty-five states that, as of March 2013, have adopted part or all the Uniform Trust Code. You can get a list at FindLaw.com that displays which part of the "titles" and "chapters" of the UTC were adopted by each state. Chances are you won't want to look any further, because the specific details of each provision of the code are mind-numbingly dense and jargon-laden.

Trustees may be unpaid, charge whatever the traffic will bear, or be paid based on the reasonable compensation section of the Uniform Trust Code. Many states apply a cap on compensation for trustees and executors. Compensation can be a flat fee, a percentage of the assets or earnings on assets, or according to work done at an hourly rate. Since some trustees actually do a fair amount of work — keeping records, filing taxes, and managing assets — sometimes the trustee compensation can be quite high.

In the end, the return on the trust's investments, business, or property belongs to the beneficiary. A trustee who dips too deeply into the trust's assets without justification is failing to perform his fiduciary duty and can be charged with a crime. Stealing from a trust is named "self-dealing," but other breaches of good faith include engaging in conflicts of interest, such as front-running the purchase of a stock for the fiduciary's personal account with the knowledge that he will be buying it for the trust the next day. Still another conflict of interest would be taking a commission for driving trust business to a particular vendor.

Violating fiduciary duty is a civil offense and often not hard to prove — you don't have to prove intent to defraud, which is actually quite difficult, but only that the fiduciary breached his position of trust for personal gain. Courts then require the fiduciary to return stolen funds and to disgorge profits even if the trust owner didn't suffer an actual loss, or damages. In some instances, a civil lawsuit against a fiduciary by the trust owner will be accompanied by a criminal case brought by the state.

Your fortune, no matter how great or small, is far too precious to be left in the hands of the state. To be sure your wishes are carried out to the letter, keep these "do's and don'ts" in mind:

DaVINCI DO'S

- To save your heirs the red tape, take the time to know your state probate laws. For smaller estates, refer to Nolo.com/legal-encyclopedia/probate-shortcuts-in-your-state-31020.html for state-by-state details.

- Although holographic (handwritten) wills are recognized in 26 states, it's always best to have an attorney draft your will. As well, do-it-yourself templates are a good starting point, but the final product should be left to a professional.

- Protect yourself or a loved one from undue influence by visiting EldersAndCourts.org/elder-abuse/key-issues/capacity-consent-and-undue-influence.aspx, (757) 259-1593.

DaVINCI DON'TS

- Never choose a trustee or executor out of obligation or guilt. Instead, pick someone you are certain will be fair, objective, and impartial.

- Do not put your assets in a living trust if you want to protect them from creditors, lawsuits, or if you are going through the divorce process. Instead, place your assets in an irrevocable trust.

- If you have had your will amended, don't forget to destroy all previous copies. Old versions could cause undue strife and even feuding among your loved ones.

Trading and Investing: Rules for Success

7

THE INTERNET IS chock-full of articles like "The Only Five Investment Rules You'll Ever Need" and "The Top Ten Investments of the Year." From the professional to the guy in the next cubicle, the sheer amount of trading or investing advice available online and otherwise can leave the best of us wondering whom to trust. The rules for success in this chapter are designed to be a wide-angle overview for beginners, while still including some useful gems for more experienced investors.

What is the difference between a trader and an investor? We think of traders as wild-eyed speculators, jumping on the latest bandwagon and therefore taking a lot of risk, while an investor is a serious guy in a pin-striped suit. These stereotypes are outdated and wrong. It's better to think of a trader as someone who buys a security with a specific price-target in mind and the intention to take profit when the target is hit, within a relatively short period of time (less than a year or two). An investor, on the other hand, is someone who buys securities deemed to have high fundamental value for a holding period with no expiration date — essentially, forever.

That is a bit of a caricature, because even long-term, buy-and-hold investor Warren Buffett sells stocks sometimes, but it serves to point out that a big, fat error lies in thinking that the holding period determines the level of risk. If the trader is using a stop-loss to protect against the risk of a price decline and is disciplined about taking profits when the target is hit, he is actually taking far less risk than the fundamentals-based investor who is operating on assumptions about "value" and actually has no money-management rules at all. A disciplined trader can be likened to a sniper, while the value-investor wields a shotgun.

So why do we persist in thinking trading is dangerous, while long-term investing is a proper place to put savings? At a guess, trading seems more dangerous because only a tiny percentage of traders do it right — with strict money management rules — and because trading seems like "speculation" or "gambling." Speculation is a dirty word in English, with deep, negative connotations, like picking which horse will win the race based on its name or the jockey's colors. But consider that speculation is actually a statistics-based undertaking of setting odds based on past performance. At its highest levels, speculation is as mathematically sophisticated as any of the hard sciences. And gambling is the exact opposite — betting on an outcome when the odds of winning are 50-50 at best (and usually less). An example is betting that after 100 coin tosses have come up heads, the next one will be tails. This is the gambler's fallacy. The coin doesn't know it came up heads 100 times. The odds of tails are still 50 percent.

Keep the idea of the disciplined trader in mind as you consider whether it's realistic to wonder if you could make a little extra money trading securities in retirement. After all, if you are near retirement or already retired, your prospects for an increase in earned income is very low or zero. Can you trade your way to a bigger rainy-day fund?

Yes, if you have aptitude and a willingness to work fairly hard — at least several hours a day.

No, if you lack intrinsic aptitude and are not willing to put in the hours.

It should be obvious that in any new endeavor, you can't expect to jump in with both feet and be successful in day one. And yet newsletter writers and other promoters try to overcome your common sense by promising surefire, fool-proof trading and investment advice. Even the rawest of novices is supposed to be able to employ some secret, magic, trading idea. But there are no secrets, no magic, and no surefire methods in trading and investing, and there is no activity that does not benefit from education and mental preparation.

Rule 1: Achieve Basic Financial Literacy

Most Americans lack basic financial literacy, according to a Securities and Exchange study published in August 2012 that was required by the Dodd-Frank Wall Street Reform and Consumer Protection Act (passed in July 2010 and still not fully implemented as of year-end 2013). The main thrust of Dodd-Frank is to improve the timing, content, and format (including plain English instead of tiny-font legalese) of disclosures to investors in financial products and services — and their providers. To figure out how to do that, the SEC was tasked with finding out what the average investor knows and does not know.

The results are shocking. The study, conducted with the Library of Congress, aptly named The Library of Congress Report, found that: Studies consistently show that American investors lack basic financial literacy. For example, studies have found that investors do not understand the most elementary financial concepts, such as compound interest and inflation.

> Moreover, many investors do not understand other key financial concepts, such as diversification or the differences between stocks and bonds, and are not fully aware of investment costs and their impact on investment returns.

> According to the Library of Congress Report, studies show that investors lack critical knowledge that would help them protect themselves from investment fraud. In particular, surveys demonstrate that certain subgroups, including women, African-Americans, Hispanics, the oldest segment of the elderly population, and those who are poorly educated, have

an even greater lock of investment knowledge than the average general population."

The Library of Congress Report concludes that 'low levels of investor literacy have serious implications for the ability of broad segments of the population to retire comfortably, particularly in an age dominated by defined-contribution retirement plans. Furthermore, it states that 'intensifying efforts to educate investors is essential,' and that investor education programs should be tailored to specific subgroups 'to maximize their effectiveness.' (SEC.gov/news/studies/2012/917-financial-literacy-study-part1.pdf.)

So, quick — what's a derivative? Explain compound interest in twenty-five words or less, and define why, exactly, diversification is a good thing.

You may think that you intend only to buy a handful of blue-chip stocks to hold permanently, so you don't need to know about derivatives or diversification. But you would be wrong. Blue-chip status is not permanent; think of once high-flying Kodak and ATT, ousted from the Dow Jones Industrial Average in 2004, or Hewlett-Packard and Bank of America, removed in 2013. Professional equity managers pare their positions in these companies, whose price always falls after they are removed from the index.

Having said that, a simple, one-time investment in a mutual fund that tracks the Dow-Jones Industrial Average or the Standard & Poor's 500 index has a far more stable price history — you will not get an unhappy surprise if one specific company or sector hits a rough patch.

A mutual fund and exchange traded fund (ETF) are index-tracking funds that have far lower price-volatility and lower transaction costs for the investor, since there isn't any real "management" going on; the choice of securities is a given by inclusion in the index. John Bogle, the inventor of index-tracking funds, puts it this way: "Don't look for the needle. Buy the haystack."

DIVIDEND STOCKS

If one does want to venture into blue-chip, dividend-paying stocks, they should look at those like Procter & Gamble and Coca-Cola — global income stocks that are not only well-positioned in the United States, but also in the four major emerging markets of Brazil, China, Russia, and India. For more on dividend-paying stocks, we encourage you to check out Jeremy Siegel's *Stocks for the Long Run*, Fifth Edition.

Buying the haystack in the form of an index-tracking fund is diversification. If one component of the index is down, another component is likely going up, hence the stable price history. That's only one form of diversification, though — you are still fully exposed to a general stock market slide into a bear market (a move down by 20 percent or more). This is sometimes named "market risk."

Should you worry about it? You bet. We have had 25 bear markets since 1929, or roughly one every 3.4 years. The average loss is 35 percent and the average length of time a bear market lasts before recovery is 10 months. The 1929 crash took over 20 years to get back to the starting point. If circumstances force you to sell your index-tracking fund before the market recovers, you face substantial losses. It goes without saying that you would have zero losses if your money were stashed in an FDIC-insured savings account.

Rule 2: It's Not Savings Unless It's a Savings Account

When it comes to savings, federally insured savings accounts and US government debt is your best bet. It's only "savings" when the money is placed in a federally insured bank account or a US government security. You are probably safe in buying the debt of AAA sovereigns, such as Australia, New Zealand, and Canada (of the thirteen AAA sovereigns in the world today), too, although that may give you a counter-productive currency risk. And many corporations are rated triple A. But in the case of other sovereigns and corporations, while your capital might be safe enough, it's not guaranteed. For US citizens, federally insured bank accounts and US government debt are as close to "guaranteed" as you can get.

That being said, we must bear in mind that the United States and other Western governments are treading on shaky budgetary ground. Huge entitlement programs and high government debt drives interest rates up, edging out private investors, which in turn causes inflation. Fixed-income investments, like Treasury bills, bonds, and notes are most affected by inflation. Investopedia.com offers this example to explain the dangers of inflation on fixed-income investments:

Suppose that a year ago you invested $1,000 in a Treasury bill with a 10% yield. Now that you are about to collect the $1,100 owed to you, is your $100 (10%) return real? Of course not! Assuming inflation was positive for the year, your purchasing power has fallen and, therefore, so has your real return. We have to take into account the chunk inflation has taken out of your return. If inflation was 4%, then your return is really 6%. As an investor, you must look at your real rate of return. Unfortunately, investors often look only at the nominal return and forget about their purchasing power altogether.

It's important to understand this savings aspect of money management, because you will read that buying ABC stock or XYZ fund is "saving." This is a misuse of the word, and can lead you astray. Most people think their pension and tax-deferred IRA's are their savings. On the whole, it's acceptable to think this way, and yet pensions are occasionally mismanaged (think of WorldCom and Enron) and if your IRA is heavily invested in speculative equities, its value is by no means assured.

If you are a disciplined trader and succeed in making good profits, the smart strategy is to "sweep" some percentage of those gains into safer savings.

Rule 3: Only Greater Risk Boosts Return

Near year-end 2013, the return on a bank savings account was less than 1 percent. The yield on a 12-month US government bill is 0.13 percent, and returns on US government paper rises from there to 0.29 percent for a 2-year note, 1.35 percent for a 5-year note, and just under three percent for a 10-year note. Meanwhile, the US equity markets are up by 20 to 30 percent. You can check these returns throughout the day, by the way, at Bloomberg.com (look for "market data").

It seems obvious that the stock market is the best place to put your money for a better return. From 1900 to 2013, the Standard & Poor's equity index has been in twenty-four bull market phases, meaning it rose over 20 percent. Each one averaged about three years, and the average return of each of the bull markets was 127.36 percent. In the thirty winning years since 1975, the S&P

TABLE 7-1: GAIN NEEDED TO RECOVER A LOSS

Loss	Gain Needed to Recover Loss
10%	11.1%
20%	25.0%
30%	42.9%
40%	66.7%
50%	100.0%
60%	150.0%
75%	300.0%

Source: Adapted from http://dshort.com/articles/2009/break-even-curve.html

went up zero to 10 percent in eight years (gaining an average of four percent), up 10 percent to 20 percent in ten years (gaining an average of 14.9 percent), and up over 20 percent in 12 years (gaining an average of 24.9 percent).

To buy and hold securities for a long period of time is a well-documented path to accumulating capital, but *only if you get in at the best time — just ahead of a bull market.* For example, from January 2000 to October 2002, the S&P fell 50 percent. If you were a die-hard buy-and-holder, you then needed to make 100 percent to get back to where you started. Ask yourself how often anyone makes a 100 percent return on investment.

You could get unlucky in your timing and risk a big chunk of your savings in a market that can crash. In 2008, the S&P lost 38.5 percent. Of the eight losing years since 1975, this was the worst one.

The stock market is not a safe, surefire way to improve return, and it isn't "easy."

Rule 4: Leverage Boosts Return But Increases Risk

You may see a promotion for a secret, 10 percent dividend, tax-free investment "backed by the US government." At a time when the rate of return on safe savings are so low, a tax-free return of 10 percent looks too good to be true.

And, of course, it is. The "secret" investment is plain, old municipal bonds bundled together and sold as a fund that makes a monthly distribution. Closed-end municipal bond funds issue a fixed number of shares and trade on an exchange like a stock, and can be priced at a premium to the underlying assets in the fund when demand is high, or at a discount when demand is low. The fund may not trade at all if it has a small number of participants, called a lack of "liquidity." In other words, the price of these funds is sensitive to interest rate changes and expected interest rate changes in the overall economy, regardless of the stated coupon yield of the original issues.

Income from municipals is indeed (generally) tax-free, but municipal bonds are not "backed by the US government." What's backed is the tax-free status. What about that wonderful 10 percent yield? It is available only through leverage, i.e., the fund borrows the money to purchase the munis. Here's how leverage works: When you put down $10 and borrow $10 to buy something for $20 and get a $1 return, your return is 10 percent even though the actual stated yield on the $20 asset is actually five percent. Borrowing half the money to make the purchases "leverages" your original amount.

This is not to say that municipal bond funds are a bad idea. Defaults among municipalities are relatively low, although they do happen (Orange County, Detroit). But the price of the closed-end, municipal fund is vulnerable to volatility when interest rates rise or are expected to rise (just like government securities, the value of these bonds depreciate rapidly in a high inflation environment). You might end up buying at a premium and needing to sell at a discount. And there is nothing inherently wrong with using leverage to boost investment returns, but if you use leverage, *you certainly want to know about it* from the beginning. The promotional hype fails to disclose that the "secret" is not municipal bond funds themselves, but the leverage used to get the high return.

When you see a promotion making overheated claims, you need to ask yourself: What's the catch? In this case, you have to sit through a promotion for an hour before getting the name of the fund, and then troll the internet for reviews and advice. The muni-bond-fund idea may or may not pass muster with your own personal risk appetite, but the point is that the promoter used trickery to lure you into buying his particular muni bond funds. He did not disclose the leverage or the possibility of price volatility that is an inherent feature of all closed-end funds. Do you really want to do business with someone who uses trickery and fails to disclose not one, but two key characteristics of the investment?

Here's where willingness to work comes into play. You need to be able to sit through the hype, be savvy enough to know the relevant questions, research the features of the promoted investment in an emotionally neutral way, look up the various leveraged muni bond funds available, and decide whether the risk is worth the reward. Depending on how much patience you have, this could take a full day, or eight hours of researching muni bond funds.

Let's say you decide in favor of buying a leveraged muni bond fund. Now you have to pick one from among the dozens available, which means researching the fund sponsor. Finally, once you have bought the fund, you need to track the sponsor's rating, and the rating and price of the fund. You can keep a handwritten log, although a spreadsheet would be more efficient. Not everyone enjoys tracking investments. Many individuals want to buy it and forget about it, and yet it's your money and your responsibility to ensure you don't have a loser that will reduce your capital. Not tracking existing investments is to violate the first rule of investing: to preserve capital.

The potential for loss in trading and investing is never zero. Every single asset into which you can place your capital that isn't an insured savings account or a US government security has some probability of failing. You can raise return over a savings account only by means of:

- increased risk
- leverage

Rule 5: Seeking Risk on Purpose

Given the low rates on risk-free assets, you will want to take some risk in order to beef up returns, but in a sensible and reasonable manner. You will see advertisements for specific investments that will return 45 percent in a year, or some other really high number. While it's perfectly true that some investments can return such high numbers, the trick is finding them ahead of the move. You have to wonder why those who claim they can do that — identify winners before they take off — would want to sell that information to you. In practice, most hucksters of trading advice will offer

TABLE 7-2: S&P PERFORMANCE 1975 TO 2012 — LOSING YEARS

No. of Years	Year	Opening Price	Closing Price	Gain/Loss	Percent Gain/Loss	Average
1	1981	135.76	122.55	-13.21	-9.73 %	
2	1990	353.4	330.22	-23.18	-6.56 %	
3	1994	466.45	459.27	-7.18	-1.54 %	
4	2000	1469.25	1320.28	-148.97	-10.14 %	
5	2001	1320.28	1148.08	-172.2	-13.04 %	
6	2002	1148.08	879.82	-268.26	-23.37 %	
7	2008	1468.36	903.25	-565.11	-38.49 %	
8	2011	1257.64	1257.6	-0.04	0.00 %	
					-102.87%	**-12.86%**

S&P PERFORMANCE 1975 TO 2012 — LOW RETURN YEARS

No. of Years	Year	Opening Price	Closing Price	Gain/Loss	Percent Gain/Loss	Average
1	1978	95.1	96.73	1.63	1.71 %	
2	1984	164.93	167.24	2.31	1.40 %	
3	1987	242.17	247.08	4.91	2.03 %	
4	1992	417.09	435.71	18.62	4.46 %	
5	1993	435.71	466.45	30.74	7.06 %	
6	2004	1111.92	1211.92	100	8.99 %	
7	2005	1211.92	1248.29	36.37	3.00 %	
8	2007	1418.3	1468.36	50.06	3.53 %	
					32.18 %	**4.02 %**

S&P PERFORMANCE 1975 TO 2012 — MEDIUM RETURN YEARS

No. of Years	Year	Opening Price	Closing Price	Gain/Loss	Percent Gain/Loss	Average
1	1976	90.19	107.46	19.15	19.15 %	
2	1979	96.73	107.94	11.21	11.59 %	
3	1982	122.55	140.64	18.09	14.76 %	
4	1983	140.64	164.93	24.29	17.27 %	
5	1986	211.28	242.17	30.89	14.62 %	
6	1988	247.08	277.72	30.64	12.40 %	
7	1999	1229.23	1469.25	240.02	19.53 %	
8	2006	1248.29	1418.3	170.01	13.62 %	
9	2010	1115.1	1257.64	142.54	12.78 %	
10	2012	1257.6	1426.19	168.59	13.41 %	
					149.13 %	**14.91 %**

No. of Years	Year	Opening Price	Closing Price	Gain/Loss	Percent Gain/Loss	Average
			S&P PERFORMANCE 1975 TO 2012 — HIGH RETURN YEARS			
1	1975	68.56	90.19	21.63	31.55 %	
2	1980	107.94	135.76	27.82	25.77 %	
3	1985	167.24	211.28	44.04	26.33 %	
4	1989	277.72	353.4	75.68	27.25 %	
5	1991	330.22	417.09	86.87	26.31 %	
6	1995	459.27	615.93	156.66	34.11 %	
7	1996	615.93	740.74	124.81	20.26 %	
8	1997	740.74	970.43	229.69	31.01 %	
9	1998	970.43	1229.23	258.8	26.67 %	
10	2003	879.82	1111.92	232.1	26.38 %	
12	2009	903.25	1115.1	211.85	23.45 %	
					299.09 %	**24.92 %**

Source: Adapted from http://www.1stock1.com/1stock1_141.htm.

twenty names and when three of them succeed in racking up a good gain, those are the only ones they advertise the following year. Sometimes the promoters are engaging in pump-and-dump, which is to promote a stock to millions of people and hope those buyers succeed in artificially inflating the price so they can themselves dump the security at a juicy profit.

This is not to say you shouldn't subscribe to newsletters, many of which are quite good. Even the questionable ones can keep you on your toes trying to figure out the true risk and reward. But be realistic in your expectations. Table 7-1 shows clusters of returns, from all-losses to medium and high returns. In the 37 years from 1975 to 2012, the S&P had eight years of dismal losses averaging 12.86 percent — from as palatable as zero to as horrible as 38.49 percent.

The S&P also had eight years of low returns averaging 4.02 percent and ten years of medium returns averaging 14.9 percent. The high-return years numbered twelve and averaged 24.92 percent. You never know in advance which cluster the upcoming year will belong to, and besides, it's unlikely that you'll buy on January 1 and sell on December 31, so measuring returns by calendar year serves only one purpose — to inject perspective into your expectations.

You may very well be able to pick up a 45 percent return on a single name, but you shouldn't count on it.

Rule 6: Avoid Catastrophic Losses, Part 1

Before placing your capital in any security, you need to ask yourself how much you are willing to lose if it turns out to be a dud. If you say you are unwilling to take any loss at all, ever, then you should not be investing in equities at all and should stick to 100 percent safe savings. If you invest in equities, you will take losses. You need to accept that, but you don't need to accept all the loss the market delivers.

The way to avoid catastrophic losses (like the 38.5 percent loss in 2008) is to use a stop-loss order. Let's say you buy Security ABC at a price of $40. You believe that that this stock has the potential to rise to $50, or a gain of 25 percent. But if you are wrong and instead it falls, you want to exit the position at a 20 percent loss, or $32.00. You tell your broker (or enter it electronically) to sell at $32.00 on a "good-'til-cancelled" (GTC) basis. In practice, the price may gap over the exact level of $32.00 and you may exit at the next available lower price, but the point is that you are actively taking the single best counter-measure to preserve capital.

Let's say the stock has now risen to $45.00, halfway to your target. You want to keep at least some of the gain, so you raise your stop to keep it a constant 20 percent of market value, or $45 minus 20 percent or $9 = $36.00. You can change this "trailing stop" as often as you wish — daily, if you have the time and energy. One virtue of a trailing stop is that it automatically gets you out of a security whose price is falling. If you didn't have the stop, you might think the falling price was just a temporary aberration. This is wishful thinking, not good money management.

Of all the tools in the trader's toolkit, the stop-loss is the absolute, number one essential. What is the best percentage to use in your stop-loss? If you are statistically minded, you would calculate the normal variance around a moving average of your stock's price, and set the stop at that number plus a little more. Prices do not move in a straight line. It might be normal for your stock to vary by as much as your stop amount ($8 or $9) on a regular basis over a short period of time, like three months. You would be getting stopped out all the time in the case just presented. A wider stop would be more convenient — or you should pick a stock with less variability. William O'Neil of *Investor's Business Daily* made the 8 percent stop-loss rule popular. Famous investor Gerald Loeb and others used a 10 percent rule. But no single number is the "right" number. Whatever percentage you pick should be appropriate to the variability of your security's price and the amount of cash in dollar terms you are willing to lose in order to get the opportunity to make your target gain — in this case, 25 percent.

If the stop-loss rule makes sense to you and you accept that you should never buy a security without one, you may have aptitude for trading and investing. Another aspect of the right mind-set is a healthy dose of skepticism about all the numbers you see and all the statements you read. This is because trading and investing are not like "earning" money by any other method. If you make a product or provide a service, the quid-pro-quo is entirely clear. But in trading and investing, your gain is always somebody else's loss. That's why it's called a zero-sum game.

For example, you think Green Widget stock is going up and you buy it at $10 per share. The seller thinks it's not going up, or at the least that $10 per share is a fair price. But Green Widget doubles to $20. You are the winner of all the gain and the seller has a $10 opportunity loss (by selling his Green Widget stock, he lost the opportunity to make that extra $10). You got the sum and he got zero. In the Green Widget transaction, there was one winner and one loser. For you to make money, somebody else has to lose. In this case, the seller may have sold Green Widget because he read a review trashing Green Widget management and products and predicting doom. But next time it could be you who reads the review and gets tricked into selling. Why would someone want to scare you into selling? Because he secretly thinks or knows it's going up, and he wants to buy more cheaply. Markets are full of smart and devious people who want to take *your* money.

And sometimes they will succeed in taking your money, usually because you made a mistake. Often that mistake could not have been avoided and can be seen only in retrospect. Take, for example, one of the star stocks of 2013: Apple — the largest US company by market value. Apple released a disappointing iPhone model on September 10 and the stock dropped from a high of $507.92 the day before, to $450.12 on September 16 (or by about 11 percent).

Let's say you couldn't tolerate a loss of over 10 percent and so you sold the stock. To have a stop-loss order is a well-accepted management technique, so no one would criticize you for taking that loss. As it happened, only a few days later on September 23, Apple released another iPhone model and the stock, already rising off the low, proceeded to $525.96 a month later.

Hard as it may be to swallow, selling after a 10 percent loss was the correct thing to do, and not really a "mistake." Over long periods of time, selling losers is a key technique for preserving capital. The point is not that you might have somehow predicted the first iPhone model would be badly received and the second model would be a winner, but that you will take losses when you trade and invest in securities. Again, if you cannot stomach any losses at all, trading securities is not for you. Good trading management seeks to make profits that are higher than the inevitable losses, not to make only profits. Having every trade be a winner is worse than unrealistic — it's delusional. Aptitude for engaging in securities trading requires a willingness to accept losses.

Rule 7: Avoid Catastrophic Losses, Part 2

The second way to avoid catastrophic losses is to diversify. Many a big fortune has been lost by concentrating all or most of the capital in a single undertaking, whether equities, a private placement/venture capital, or real estate. Diversification reduces risk. The core idea is that events that have a negative effect on one security or class of securities will have a positive effect on a different class, and a properly organized portfolio of non-correlated securities will generate the greatest return for the least risk along a curve. You can choose your mix of risk and return from the curve depending on your appetite for risk. In practice, most people don't know their appetite for risk until they experience too much risk (losses) or regret at opportunities lost.

Diversification doesn't mean any old random collection of seemingly unrelated securities — the asset classes need to be actually non-correlated with one another. Obviously, you don't get diversification from buying Big Pharmaceutical Company A and Big Pharmaceutical Company B, but you may not get diversification from Big Pharmaceutical Company A plus Big Airline B, either. In this instance it's the "Big" part that counts — large-cap stocks tend to have some correlation with one another, and to be relatively non-correlated with small cap stocks.

Asset classes are generally divided into large- and small-company equities, equity and fixed income, different types of commodities (metals vs. grains), and so on; but classification doesn't necessarily tell you how closely correlated or uncorrelated any two securities might be. Besides, we need to add another factor — not only the highest return for the least risk, but also stability of returns. It may seem too obvious to mention, but you can have an optimum mix of risk and return on a theoretical basis, but still get disappointing results if your entry-level is bad. In other words, if you buy at the top of a market that then falls, you may have the right mix but still end up with a sub-par return because you selected your securities based on past returns and had a false expectation that the same would hold in the future. Alas, the future never repeats exactly.

REIT DIVERSIFICATION

To diversify even further, consider the Real Estate Investment Trust (REIT). Few can afford to purchase an array of income producing and commercial real estate. In steps the REIT — shares of real estate equity that trade just like stocks (often called "real estate stocks"), which allow you to own interest in commercial and investment properties with limited risk.

You can see optimum portfolio allocations online from numerous universities. You can even see demonstrations on portfolio allocation on YouTube (YouTube.com/watch?v=Rz5tGZdyViw). Don't be intimidated. You will hear of systematic risk vs. non-systematic risk, and other initially mind-boggling concepts. But your intuitive understanding that diversification reduces risk is a perfectly good starting point. Once you know what to look for, you can search online for the portfolio allocation advice that you can understand. You don't need to know how to apply quadratic equations to get risk and return estimates from just about every brokerage site. Vanguard, for example, shows the riskiness of each sector and fund. Morningstar details how adding some mid-size and small-cap stocks provide greater return without adding risk, so if you were thinking only of large-cap, blue-chips, you might want to think again.

You don't need to get into the heavy nitty-gritty of optimum portfolio allocation, but you should make an effort to ensure you are not overly concentrated in only one or two assets classes or several asset classes that are highly correlated. In addition to brokerage sites, many online resources offer tables of correlations, including AssetCorrelation.com, among others.

Rule 8: Learn to Look at Charts

You will see analysts deriding chart-reading as worthless and dangerous. In contrast, proponents think chart-reading beats trying to understand all the fundamentals of any security, which can be immensely complex and are, in any case, subject to the whims of the overall market index to which they belong. As much as 25 percent of the price of a stock is due to what the index is doing, so if there is a panic or a crash, even the bluest of blue chips is going to move in lockstep. This is named the "falling tide lowers all boats" concept.

You don't have to become a full-fledged market timer to apply a few common sense charting rules. Let's say you like Security XYZ, and you pull up a chart on your broker's website or any of the free sites like StockCharts.com, Finance.Yahoo.com, or BarCharts.com. You see that XYZ is falling and has been falling for many months. It's below its 50-day and 200-day moving average. You may be sold on this name, but it's logical to wait to buy it until it has stopped falling. To figure that out, you can look at simple indicators or just eyeball it. If you have the time and aptitude, learning a few indicators is not hard and can contribute to your bottom line by keeping you out of still-falling securities or identifying promising names that have already bottomed.

The ranks of technical analysis traders have ballooned in recent years, including the many retirees who have become the bedrock of advisory subscription services. Technical analysis, or chart-reading, has actually been around since the turn of the twentieth century, and was described in the first instance by Charles Dow, a founder of the *Wall Street Journal*. Dow observed that when the transport stocks (initially railroads) were rising, it meant the overall economy (and thus corporate earnings) was robust, and so the overall index tended to rise, too. Dow also observed that stock prices don't move in straight lines, but directionally trended with regular pullbacks. Over the years, technical methods evolved — and very rapidly since the advent of the PC — to include not only the familiar moving averages and momentum metrics, but also numerous arithmetic rejiggerings of price and volume to try to detect the market's sentiment.

To know at least a little about technical analysis is a defensive move if you decide to embark on securities trading to supplement your retirement income — you need to know what many other people in the market are thinking in order to decide whether you want to go with the crowd or fight against it.

Rule 9: Conventional Wisdom is (Probably) Bunk

Very little of the advice you see from financial professionals or promoters is useful. A "rule" that is useful and true in one context is just plain wrong in a different context. Some advisors say always pick stocks that deliver dividends, while others say never pick stocks with dividends because they underperform the broad market. Neither advice is true and correct in all circumstances. Some advisors promote one sector over another, depending on the business cycle (sector rotation), and some like value over growth (or growth over value). There is no single, best way to pick stocks, although William O'Neil's CAN SLIM approach, from his book *How to Make Money in Stocks* continues to stand the test of time.

One of the most perfidious "rules" of investing is that you should be taking more risk when you are young and have more years of earning ahead, so that a 30-year old should have a high percentage of his capital in equities, while a retiree should have very little. If you hire an investment advisor when you are 55 and older, he is sure to show you how to reallocate your capital to reduce risk. After all, your earning years are behind you, or nearly so, and so is your ability to save up more capital in the event of a big loss. A portfolio allocation of 60 percent stocks and 40 percent bonds that is "appropriate" for a 40-year old is shifted to 10-20 percent equities and 80-90 percent bonds for those over 55.

Evidently investment advisors have never heard of the stop-loss order, nor do they think that by the time you are 55 and older, it's possible your judgment is sounder than when you were 30 or 40. If you are already retired, you would have the time to research

> **CAN SLIM**
>
> **CAN SLIM**, the brainchild *Investor's Business Daily* Co-Founder William O'Neil, is a successful investment strategy popularized by his book, *How to Make Money in Stocks*. This mnemonic device/acronym stands for: **C**urrent Earnings; **A**nnual Earnings; Something **N**ew; **S**upply and Demand; **L**eader or **L**aggard; **I**nstitutional Sponsorship; and **M**arket Direction. If certain criteria are met by a company in each category, it's stocks are almost guaranteed to be profitable.

investments and have the life-experience to winnow the wheat from the chaff. A hard-and-fast rule that puts 80 percent of your portfolio in safe, government bonds *because of your age* is basically depriving you of the chance to build capital. Of course, some people lack the aptitude to engage in trading and investing at any age, but it should be up to you — not some whippersnapper investment advisor — to determine the mix of safe and risky assets. Portfolio optimization programs should be built on financial literacy, brainpower, and expertise — not age.

Another piece of conventional wisdom embedded in investment advisor plans and programs is that you should place your funds in asset classes that have performed well over the past three or five years. When a market has a negative return in that period, it gets removed from the list of available securities and asset classes altogether. But market lore has it that the best time to buy is when there is blood in the streets — i.e., a crash has already occurred and whatever remains standing will go up to pre-crash levels. After the Asian crisis crash of 1997-98, for example, the stock markets of all the affected countries (Thailand, Hong Kong, Malaysia, Indonesia, et al.) were off-limits to investors trying to put together a globally diversified portfolio. But over the next decade, those were the markets that outperformed all other markets. The US market crashed 38.5 percent in 2008, and yet "home country bias" kept most investors in the US markets when diversification to foreign markets, especially in high-risk emerging markets, would have outperformed the US equity market over the next three years.

Rule 10: Options

Options are financial derivatives that grow more popular with every passing year. The reason options became so popular is a tactic named the "covered call." This strategy entails selling someone else the right to buy a security that you own at some point of time in the future for a price higher than today's price. In return, the buyer pays you a small amount of money, named a premium, for the right (but not the obligation) to buy the security from you. Since you already own the security, the call option you are selling is "covered" — you don't have to rush out to buy it in order to deliver to the buyers if the option gets "called." Be sure to read on for the "naked" option — when you don't already own the security but sell a call option on it.

The first advantage of a covered call is that you get to keep the premium no matter what happens afterwards. If the buyer exercises his right to buy the security from you, the amount of the premium is not subtracted from the amount of money you receive on the sale. If the option expires worthless, you still get to keep the premium. In sum, you get to have your cake and eat it too — you get cash money today while still owning the stock. Better yet, you know the target price at which you will be selling if the price goes up and reaches the strike price so that the buyer is likely to exercise the option. To sell a covered call is to set a profit target. Along with the stop-loss, profit-targeting is critical to "planning the trade" — a key component of good money management.

An example of a covered call is owning a stock now worth $50 that you project will go to $60 in a year, or a gain of 20 percent. But you would be willing to settle for a sale at $55 in six months. If you sell a call option at $55, you will receive a premium of, say, $3 per share (6 percent), or $300 on a security that cost you $5,000. Now the price does indeed go to $55 (or a little more), the buyer exercises his option, and you are forced to sell at $55.00. You are losing the opportunity embodied in the now higher price, but you are getting $55 + $3, or $58 per share, giving you $5,800 for something that cost $5,000, or a return of 16 percent — and in six months. If the stock persists in rising and doubles to $100, you have the 16 percent cash gain, but a $42 opportunity loss — the extra amount you would have made if your stock had not been called away from you.

If the price falls to $40 instead of rising and the call option buyer is not likely to buy from you, you still own the stock. Your true loss is not $10, though, but rather $10 minus the $3 premium you collected. If you were using a 20 percent stop-loss number that would normally have had you exit the security at $40, you could lower the stop to $37. But in practice, you wouldn't want to sell at $40 or $37, because then you would be "naked" and have to buy the security fast if the price reversed back to the upside. People always imagine they will remember to do that, but can easily get blindsided by a runaway rally. The better course of action if you want to sell the stock at $37 is to buy back the call option you sold earlier, which is now cheaper.

Covered calls are a way to add to returns if prices move up, and to reduce losses if prices move down. The only drawback is limiting upside gain — although nothing is stopping you from buying another set of shares of the same security on which you do not sell a call. You could create your own drawback by selling a security on which you have written calls and thus going "naked," but that is human error and not a risk intrinsic to options. Writing a covered call is like getting a dividend from a stock that otherwise doesn't offer a dividend. In addition, the income from call options reduces the risk of a portfolio by lowering the cost basis.

You can even buy into a mutual fund that specializes in writing covered calls. If writing covered calls is a no-lose situation, why isn't everyone doing it? Plenty of people do continue to write covered calls, of course, but many become discouraged by the skimpy premiums available for "out-of-the-money calls" (the profitable ones where the strike price is higher than the current price). Instead of getting $3 for the $55 strike call option described, for example, the premium may be only 85¢. Eight-five cents doesn't go very far in reducing your cost basis, and to take in $85 on 100 shares costing $5,000 is a return of only 1.7 percent.

Besides, in a raging bull market like the 2013 market, you would have been called on everything and missed opportunities left and right, while getting what in hindsight is inadequate compensation. A third drawback is that the learning curve for option pricing is very steep. You have to juggle the strike price, expiration date, and premium, which entail an understanding of net present value, among other complexities. Some options price charts are almost impossible to read. One that is more accessible is BornToSell .com/covered-call-scanner, which shows you almost one thousand names and the associated return *if the market is flat*. But in general, once you start learning about options, the more complex you realize it is and how much mathematical skill you really should have. Options can be very intimidating.

Option basics are fairly simple, although before you know it, you have two or three moving targets all at once — real prices changing against the strike price, the overall market moving up or down, etc. Here are some general guidelines.

If you buy a "call" for a small premium, you are getting a contract that allows you to buy a security at a fixed price that you name at some future point in time. Let's say the Abracadabra Company is currently priced at $10 and you believe from research that it will double within six months. You are willing to pay $250 for the right to buy 100 shares anytime during the next six months at $15 (the "strike" price) with the idea of selling it when it gets to a higher price. The call option gives you the right, but not the obligation, to buy at $15.

Let's say the price goes to $18. Technically, you could exercise your option, buy the stock for $15, and pocket the extra $3. But you paid $250 for the option, so in fact your profit is only 50¢ per share, or $50. But you made $50 on a capital cost of $250 or 20 percent in six months, a very high return when the return on a savings account is one percent. In practice, the price of the option is keeping pace with the stock price, so you wouldn't go through the folderol of actually exercising the option, buying the stock, and then selling it — you'd simply sell the option itself. Your option went "in the money" when the price of the security rose above the strike price and it reached your breakeven when it reached the strike price plus the cost of the premium, or $17.50 per share.

What if the Abracadabra Company fails and the stock falls to $1? You let your option expire. You made a bet costing $250 on a horse that fell at the first fence. You lose it all. But it makes more sense to lose $250 on a worthless option than to lose $900, the cost of 100 shares at $10 per share at the starting point minus the $1 it's worth at the ending point.

Similarly, you can buy a "put" on a stock you are convinced will fall in price, for example, Enron. Again, you pay a premium to get the right to sell the stock at a fixed price in the future. If the stock rises, you are out of luck and you let the option expire, but if the price falls by more than the equivalent premium you paid, you will have a profit.

Here's the critical rule: As long as you are the buyer of an option, either the call or the put, the amount you can lose is limited by the cost of the premium. Technically, the amount you can make is unlimited — Abracadabra could go to $100 and you have the right to buy it for $15! In practice, prices hardly ever go from $10 to $100, so it's wise to have a sensible, price-history-based idea of potential gain.

When you become the seller of the option, called the writer, however, your risk can potentially rise to infinity. Pretend you were the writer of the Abracadabra call, not the buyer. And you don't own the stock — you are "naked." You forget that you made $250 writing the call until the broker telephones you with the news that the call-buyer wants to exercise his right to buy the stock from you. The price is now $18. You have to run out and buy the stock in order to deliver it to the buyer, costing you $1,800 minus the $250 premium or $1,550. Or alternatively, you can just buy the option back, but the price now incorporates the amount by which it's "in the money." The mistake is expensive no matter which way you resolve it to meet your contractual obligation.

Writing puts has an equivalent potential risk. When you sell a put, you are letting the buyer "put" the stock to you at a lower price. Say the current price is $12.50 and the strike price is $7.50. You collect the premium and forget about it — after all, the market is going up, not down. But as the strike date approaches, the price is falling toward the strike price and then under it, to $6.50. The buyer has the right to put the shares to you at a price of $7.50 and you are obligated by the option contract to buy them at that price, even though you could get them more cheaply in the open market. If you like the stock at any price, you end up having overpaid for it, but if you don't have the $750 at all, you have to borrow it from somewhere or your name is mud with the broker. And it gets worse if you wrote a naked put at a very high price that you think could never happen . . . until it does, like the price of gold in the week after 9/11.

Bottom line: Buying options is fairly safe, while selling them can be very dangerous unless you are covered. Options are both simple and complex — you can devise clever ways to avoid unacceptable losses on your portfolio and make a little extra return while you are at it, but to do it properly, you need to be able to evaluate the time value of the premium, alternative return on a different use of the money you put into the premium, how premiums are calculated (which involves the volatility of the stock price as well as time value), and the effort to keep it all straight and shipshape.

You know that options can be tricky when you notice that all the paperwork surrounding options comes with this disclaimer:

Options involve risks and are not suitable for everyone. Option trading can be speculative in nature and carry substantial risk of loss. Only invest with risk capital.

In other words, unless you are selling covered calls, don't put money into options that you can't afford to lose — it should be play money, not the mortgage payment. If you are methodical and mathematically adept, options may be for you — but get educated first. A good place to start is the Options Clearing Corporation's basic book, *Characteristics and Risks of Standardized Options* (OptionsClearing.com). The Securities and Exchange Commission and several exchanges have tutorials, and there is even a site named OptionTradingpedia.com. You will see many magazine articles about the opportunities inherent in trading options — after all, you seem to have control over hundreds of shares while paying only a small premium for each foray. If the concept of the time value of money eludes you, options are probably not for you.

Rule 11: Avoid Fraud and Scams

The press is full of warnings against scams — many of them targeting older people and most of them involving cyber-crime — tricking you into giving out a credit card number, Social Security number, or prepaying to get a lottery winning or inheritance. If you fell for any of these scams, or sent money to Nigeria, you should get someone else to manage your money for you.

The best rule is the old rule: If it sounds too good to be true, it is.

The cable channel CNBC has a series titled *American Greed: Scams, Schemes, and Broken Dreams,* that is well worth the time. You see charming scammers and swindlers and the tricks they use on ordinary people, as well as stars and celebrities. The lessons to be learned are many, but a summary would include:

- The swindler represents a big, legitimate organization with a long track record.

- The swindler is your friend and pretends to want what's in your best interest.

- The opportunity will get away if you don't hand over money immediately, so there is no formal documentation.

- The urgency means the swindler will take a credit card or make a visit to pick up money.

- The swindler downplays risk.

- The swindler offers something for free.

- The swindler is offering a deal over the phone or on the Internet.

You should ask for written documentation of the investment promoter's credentials, deal only with licensed and registered persons, and demand written proposals that are also registered with one or another regulator. You need to take the time to check all these licenses and registrations. In addition to checking the promoter's bona fides, keep in mind that any deal that must be done right away, with great urgency or the opportunity will be lost, is always fishy. If it's a really good opportunity, it will still be there tomorrow — good opportunities do not vanish in a puff of smoke.

REVIEW STATEMENTS

Always be sure to look closely at your statements. Any legitimate money manager will be using third-party providers like Fidelity or Schwab — the statements should come from them, and only be passed along by your money manager.

The North American Securities Administrators Association (NASAA.org) lists the top ten investor threats of the year. Some are new and some are "persistent," meaning enough people fall for them that they keep going for years. Here are some of them:

Real Estate Investment Schemes tend to focus on new developments or pooling distressed properties for renovation and flipping. Since everyone knows something about the real estate bust and evolving recovery, real estate schemes sound like a no-brainer. But "In the latest NASAA enforcement survey, real estate investments were the second-most common product leading to securities fraud investigations by state securities regulators." Researching things like title ownership, mortgage ownership, and market value takes investment savvy and a keen eye for detail. It's easy to get cheated into investing in real property where the ownerships is a complete muddle and the property is mortgaged far beyond its value.

Private Placements that escape registration requirements are the number one danger. The private placement sounds grand, but is really for investment in a business that does not exist or is advertised as substantial, but often no more than a post office box. Promotional materials may show photos of real estate and offices not owned by the private placement promoter, and other misrepresentations. Valid private placements do exist, but are for only the most sophisticated investors who have the time and money to verify the offering documents. If you are a small investor without the resources to investigate a private placement thoroughly, you should stick to registered securities that come under the regulatory purview of government agencies.

Fraudsters Using Self-Directed IRAs to Mask Deceptive Practices: Scam artists use self-directed IRAs and sometimes offer to become the custodian and trustee, which only delays discovery that the investments selected are fraudulent. Fear of triggering penalties and taxes on early withdrawals keeps the investor passive and once the scammer has you in his orbit, he may employ sheer sales skill to talk you into improper investments in real estate, precious metals, and private placements.

High-Yield Investment and Ponzi Schemes: If the return on an investment is unbelievably high and also promoted as low risk, don't believe it, however plausible the scenario. Promoters often claim affiliation with a trusted group or a background that involves an Ivy League education and running big companies with high-falutin' names. In today's information-saturated, Internet-enabled world, there is no excuse for not investigating the background of any high-yield promoter. The NASAA writes, "One way to protect yourself is to ask questions, and when you think you have asked all the questions you have, ask more questions. As Bernie Madoff, the king of Ponzi schemes, once said, he only turned people away when they asked too many questions."

Affinity Fraud is a subset of high-yield and Ponzi-scheme fraud. You think you can trust a fellow member of your church, ethnic group, or special interest group. The idea is that you let your guard down because you have a common interest with the promoter.

Risky Oil and Gas Drilling Programs: Oil and gas drilling may appear lucrative but can also carry high risk, including the risk of losing everything. You can buy into the energy sector without buying into a specific program. "There are active investigations into suspect oil and gas investment programs in more than two dozen states and in every region of the US and Canada."

Digital Currency: Virtual money like Bitcoins is an accident waiting to happen. Avoid Bitcoins and any other virtual currencies like the plague. You will have no recourse if the price falls to zero. Skepticism about the value of government-issued money is no excuse for falling for this giant, global scam.

Proxy Trading Accounts: Unlicensed persons who claim investment expertise and a great track record offer to set up or manage your existing brokerage account on your behalf. Don't do it. You will probably see large trading losses or substantial withdrawals amounting to theft. We have state and federal regulatory agencies that license and police investment professionals, who must conform to standards of ethical behavior. You can consult these regulators to make sure any advisor or manager you may be interested in hiring is licensed and registered.

You can see other tips and news about scams directed specifically to seniors at the NASAA "senior investor resource center." (NASAA.org/1723/senior-investor-resource-center/.)

Avoiding Bad Investments: Advice from Credit Analysts

It's true that making a loan at a bank is different in many ways from making an investment in a regulated market, but yet these rules are really good guides, especially for newcomers to the investment world. An easy-to-remember mantra, the "Five Ps" are fool-proof rules you should learn by heart.

People: Are the people involved honest and trustworthy? Did they ever default and decamp so there are gaps in their business history? Do you know the facts — for sure — about their background? One lie disqualifies the person permanently.

Purpose: What is the purpose of the investment? In a loan, we ask what the money is going to be used for — constructing a new office building or purchasing inventory? In investments, our purpose is always to get a return that is better than the risk-free return, but without taking too much risk. How confident are you that your choice of investment will deliver that return? Did the same investment deliver returns in the past and were they consistent over time?

Payment: How will you get repaid? What is the cash-flow or asset base that will induce other investors to support the security, or what are the supply and demand dynamics in the case of real property and commodities?

Protection: In a bank loan, protection often takes the form of collateral — assets of value laid on the line to be taken over if the borrowers fails to repay the loan. In scam investments, the promoter often says the investment is "guaranteed." Actually, very little is guaranteed under US law without qualification. Lawyers quarrel at length about what is a valid guarantee and what is a warranty or indemnification. The only investment that is well and truly guaranteed is a US government bill, note, or bond. If a promoter tells you something is guaranteed, remind him that a true guarantee should be evidenced by a signed and dated document by *the guarantor.*

What protection does the investor have against fraud and failure? When you buy regulated securities from regulated, licensed operators, you have some protection against loss and fraud by the broker and the manager of the security itself. When company management and regulators fail, as they did in the case of Enron and Refco, you can still face 100 percent loss of capital, but systemic failure like this is rare.

Perspective: How much of your savings should you put into this sector or that one, or how much into precious metals or real estate? In a nutshell, do you have a harmonious balance of investments that does not put your savings at excessive risk and allows you sleep at night?

Profitable investing requires not only risk capital, but research, patience, realism, and diligence. Try following these "do's and don'ts" to begin building a successful and well-rounded investment portfolio:

DaVINCI DO'S

- Achieve basic financial literacy. With the Internet as a resource, or even your local library, there's no excuse not to have a basic knowledge of investment instruments and jargon. Investopedia.com is an invaluable tool to get you on your way to "talking the talk" and "walking the walk."

- Once you become comfortable with the basics, begin learning to use technical analysis tools, or chart reading. This is a quick and efficient way to stay on top of market trends.

- Savings accounts and Treasury bills, bonds, notes are your safest investment options, but always remember to look at your real rate of return, which is affected by declining purchasing power via inflation. Municipal bonds should be assessed similarly.

DaVINCI DON'TS

- Don't forget the two rules of avoiding catastrophic losses: (1) Being as practical as possible, determine how much you are willing to lose should your investment tank; and (2) A properly diversified portfolio's losses will be considerably offset by its gains.

- Do not become complacent when it comes to tracking your investments. This is key to preserving capital, which, after all, is the name of the game.

- Don't be drawn into the misconception that an investment's holding period determines its level of risk. This is why stop-loss protections were invented — to protect traders against excessive price declines.

Financial Planning

8

RETIREMENT PLANNING HAS become an industry in its own right, although a formidable 40 percentof those nearing retirement decide not to use an advisor. Because retirement is such a big deal, this is puzzling. Neglecting to plan can easily mean misery in your golden years, with perpetual money worries that take all the joy out of being retired. So why do people avoid getting planning advice?

- They can't afford an advisor.

- They are ashamed about having saved so little.

- They are embarrassed about being financially illiterate.

- They think the advisor just wants to sell them financial products they won't understand or that may not be sound investments.

- They don't want to take the trouble to learn about finance.

- They don't like or trust the planning process.

Notice that nearly all these objections to using a retirement advisor are about the retiree and not about the retirement planning industry. One suspicion is well-founded: Financial service companies want to sell you products. When you do an internet search for "retirement advisors," you get almost 40 million results. The names of the organizations sound good —Retirement Advisors of America, Golden Retirement Advisors, and so on — but before long you realize these are fee-based advisors, and they don't disclose the fees until you give them your name and personal information, plus listen to their sales pitch.

An old insurance company motto is that there are five basic reasons for not making a sale: no need, no money, no trust, no hurry, and no desire. Obviously when you lose trust on your very first foray into the subject of retirement planning because it seems like these companies are out to trick you into buying something, you halt the whole process. This is a mistake, because even if you end up buying nothing from a retirement advisor, you can use the process of researching retirement planning to get educated. All advisors, including those sponsored by banks and brokers, offer seminars, webinars, and sometimes presentations that literally include a free lunch. And you should learn to overcome the "no trust" aspect because you do have a need, and depending on how far along you are in the retirement process, you may have to hurry. As for "no money," that's your own business. Nobody can force you to disclose your income or savings (except the IRS).

If you think about it, you have to overcome the same obstacles when you go to buy a new car. You know the salesman will manipulate you into disclosing facts about yourself that you don't normally tell a stranger, including how much money you have to spend. He creates a bubble of forced friendship, pretends a deal has to be done right away or the specific car you like will get snatched up, and is probably lying when he says the discount he's offering is the absolute lowest he can go. Everybody dreads the process of buying a new car because we assume the salesman is out to get us, but the secret to getting a good deal is to be prepared. You research ahead of time, and walk onto the lot with confidence.

Navigating the world of investments and retirement planning should be treated the same way you'd treat any major purchase. Yes, retirement advisors do offer a great deal of free education, but not much, if anything, in life is free. You have to sit through hours of promotional material and may have to put up with intrusive questionnaires and a fair amount of infuriating condescension in order to get cold, hard facts. But just as you need to be prepared to deal with the car salesman and his tricks of the trade, you can become prepared to deal with the retirement advisory industry.

Planning vs. Advising

The first step is to recognize that a retirement planner is not the same thing as an investment advisor. A planner covers the entire universe of retirement issues, while an advisor manages the funds you place with him. The distinction is not a clear, hard line, though, because some planners are also investment managers. A planner will help you determine:

- What your monthly income will be after you retire

- When to take Social Security benefits and how to choose a pension distribution plan

- How to minimize taxes by rearranging your investment accounts (IRA vs. Roth, for example)

- How to minimize taxes when taking withdrawals from existing accounts

- If you should pay off your mortgage before retirement and whether a reverse mortgage is a good plan for you

- Whether to keep your life insurance policies, or buy an annuity or a long-term healthcare policy

Retirement planners may charge an hourly fee or a flat, one-time fee, sometimes on a retainer basis (quarterly or annually). Those who also manage your funds will charge a percentage on the assets you place with them and also collect a commission from the financial services companies for financial products you buy from them.

A retirement advisor is a subset of the financial advisory industry, and may or may not be qualified to cover all the non-investment aspects of retirement, like minimizing taxes, reverse mortgages, and your overall portfolio.

Credentials

You will see a barrage of credential abbreviations after the names of certified and registered planners. You don't have to learn what each of them means, but it's a good idea to choose a planner that has training and certification, even if some of the certificates are fairly easy to qualify for.

An emerging credential for a retirement planner is membership in the Retirement Income Industry Association, or RIIA, founded in 2006 and offering certification in Retirement Management Analysis. The RIIA offers an online planner by state (InvestmentAdvisorChannel.com/advisor-database), but as with other such sites, you have to sign up and disclose information about yourself, such as current available assets, and you'll be asked to agree to have your information shared with potential advisors. To begin planning, visit RIIA-USA.org/consumer, or call (617) 342-7390.

For general financial planning, the top credential is Certified Financial Planner, or CFP, a certification issued by the Financial Planning Association. Again, you need to disclose your household income and investible assets in order to get a list of planners in your area. Visit the FPA website at FPAnet.org/PlannerSearch/PlannerSearch.aspx,or contact the association by phone at (800) 322-4237.

The one site that delivers actual names of certified planners in your area is BoomeRater.com. Some of the advisors are independent and some are employees or affiliated with a financial institution (broker or insurance company), and they have paid to have their name and photo included in the BoomeRater site, but they come right out and tell you the minimum income and asset level they will accept, and they list their licenses and certifications. Some have no minimum and offer a free initial consultation. BoomeRater .com also has informative articles on a range of subjects (housing, shopping, travel, etc.). To locate an advisor by zip code, visit BoomeRater.com/financial/find-a-financial-advisor.

If you are already saturated with the incomprehensible, alphabet soup of credentials, here's a sample listing from BoomeRater.com of one advisor, whose areas of expertise include:

- Elder Issues (long-term care, pre-mortem planning)

- Life Planning

- Portfolio Management

- Retirement Planning

- Securities

- Stocks and Bonds

- Tax Planning

Education and professional training includes:

- Certified Financial Planner (CFP)

- Certified in Long Term Care (CLTC)

- Registered Investment Advisor Agent

- Insurance Licensed for Life, Health, Accident, Variable Annuities in [State]

- Society of Plan Administrators and Record-keepers (SPARK) Certified Trainer

- American Society of Pension Professionals & Actuaries (ASPPA)

- BS International Business (summa cum laude), [Name] College

This particular advisor has no minimums for household income or assets, and offers a free, initial consultation. Do all these credentials add up to a trustworthy person? You can't judge trustworthiness from certifications, some of which are fairly easy to acquire, although actuarial and accounting licenses take a great deal of study. You can check out whether a planner has received any complaints at FP.net/about-cfp-board/ethics-enforcement/report-misconduct, or by calling (800) 487-1497.

The National Association of Personal Financial Advisors (NAPFA.org, 888-FEE-ONLY) has only fee-based advisors and claims independence from sellers of financial products, plus its continuing education requirement (60 hours every two years) gives its members an edge. Again, you may run into minimum asset requirements (generally $500,000). The website offers the names and information about advisors by zip code.

GarrettPlanningNetwork.com, (913) 268-1500, is another source for fee-based advisors, and in this case, you fill out a questionnaire and the company selects a few advisors for your consideration.

PaladinRegistry.com, (916) 253-3334, also matches you up with a few advisors after you fill out a questionnaire. The Paladin site has several how-to articles and other material of interest, but again, you have to disclose personal financial information to get started.

One thing you will find in the promotional material for advisors is that they offer "objective advice." But in the real financial world, there is very little objectivity. A planner may be able to nail down the optimum IRA withdrawal schedule to minimize taxes, to be sure, but nearly everything not tax-related is subject to context and preference. But to the hammer, everything looks like a nail. In other words, to a financial advisor who makes most of his income selling mutual funds, mutual funds are always the best investment vehicle. And yet you will find plenty of investment gurus who assert, credibly and at length, that mutual funds are a bad investment and exchange-traded funds (ETFs) are less costly.

One strategy previously mentioned briefly, if you have the time and the stomach for it, is to research several advisors. Attend the seminars/webinars, read the how-to booklets, check out backgrounds, discover the costs, and so on. You may still decide not to hire an advisor, but at least you will have gained an appreciation of the scope of what your plan should look like. You still need a plan and you still need to write it down, but if you are financially literate, you can do it yourself.

Do Your Homework

An advisor's credentials are no guarantee that he or she is not a crook, but it's a start. If you find an advisor you like, be careful to verify that he has some credentials, and don't just take his word for it. Incompetents and scammers alike can be charming and convincing. But in some cases, credentials have no meaning at all, unfortunately. A series of articles in *The New York Times* entitled "A Vulnerable Age" points out various ways that advisors mislead seniors into catastrophic financial errors while lining their own pockets. For example, the Veterans Administration offers accreditation to some 20,000 advisors, but the process is hardly reliable:

> The VA accreditation process is so lax that applicants provide their own background information, including any criminal records. But the VA has only four full-time employees evaluating the approximately 5,000 applications that it receives annually. Once people get the VA's stamp of approval, they rarely lose it, even if a customer complains or regulatory actions mount. Last year, the VA revoked its accreditation for two of its more than 20,000 advisers.
>
> Lawyers, financial advisers and insurance brokers have formed a lucrative alliance with retirement communities and assisted living facilities to extract many billions of taxpayer dollars from the VA, according to interviews with state and federal authorities, as well as a review by *The New York Times* of hundreds of legal documents and client contracts.
>
> Questionable actors are capitalizing on loose oversight to unlock the VA money and enrich themselves, sometimes at veterans' expense. Some advisers sell financial products like annuities and trusts that are meant to mask veterans' assets or income — arrangements can tie up family money for years or even decades. Others circumvent VA rules and charge hundreds or even thousands of dollars for advice that may — or may not — help veterans qualify. Still others offer to train lawyers and advisers about the workings of the VA.

You can find this article and others in the series at NYTimes.com/2013/12/24/business/winning-veterans-trust-and-profiting-from-it.html?hp&_r=0.

It is true that the VA offers a Veterans Pension program, but the income cut-off is $12,465 annually for a single applicant, while the average Social Security benefit is more than that. You can easily check the terms and conditions at the Veterans Affairs website

(VA.gov/explore/pensions.asp, 800-827-1000) as well as get the application forms.

A second red light is when an advisor tries to sell you plans for trusts, annuities, or other financial products designed to conceal your income or assets. While deferring and minimizing taxes is perfectly legal, when the sole intent is to hide income and assets in order to get a government benefit, your advisor is leading you into fraud. The VA doesn't track you down and take you to court for fraud, it just denies your application, but the consequences with the IRS may be more dire. The sad stories in the newspaper about veterans and their families being led astray fail to mention that (1) they could have done their homework with easily-accessible internet resources, and (2) they were seeking something that was too good to be true.

Another scam is an "advance" against a pension offered by non-bank entities that claim to be "pension advisors." A pensioner may be offered a $10,000 advance to be repaid with, say, $350 per month over five years. Because it's an advance and not a "loan," the entity avoids coming under state and federal usury laws. Do the math: $350 per month over five years equals a total cumulative payment of $21,000.

> A review by *The New York Times* of more than two dozen contracts for pension-based loans found that after factoring in various fees, the effective interest rates ranged from 27 percent to 106 percent — information not disclosed in the ads or in the contracts themselves. Furthermore, to qualify for one of the loans, borrowers are sometimes required to take out a life insurance policy that names the lender as the sole beneficiary. (NYTimes.com/2013/04/28/business/economy/pension-loans-drive-retirees-into-more-debt.html?pagewanted=all&_r=0.)

You can sign up for the AARP's Fraud Watch Network at AARP.org/money/scams-fraud/fraud-watch-network, and you can also read about scams at the FBI website, FBI.gov/scams-safety/fraud/seniors. The FBI also has a general section on scams and frauds (FBI.gov/scams-safety/fraud/fraud) that lists the usual Nigerian-letter scam and advance-fee scams, but some others you may never have heard of, like "US Treasury Direct Accounts" (which do not exist).

Retirement Investment Mentors

The problem with doing it yourself is that it can become a piece-meal project, instead of a do-it-once project that lets you move on to other things. Whether you are doing it piecemeal or all at once, though, one resource you should check is the "retirement mentors" at various sites, most of whom also have books on retirement finance to their names.

The retirement section of MarketWatch.com often has investment advice from long-time advisors, including Paul Merriman, author of delightfully titled booklets like *Get Smart or Get Screwed: How to Select and Get the Best from Your Financial Advisor*, and several how-to investing books.

Merriman says that being cheap and thinking that an investment advisor is a waste of money is a false economy. It's always smart to get a second opinion on specific things and also to get someone with fresh eyes to look at your big picture. The advisor may see that you are over-invested in a high-risk sector, without a proper appreciation of the damage it will do to your total portfolio if it were to crash. In other words, an outsider can distinguish between your wishful thinking and financial reality. For a few hundred dollars, you can get the unbiased, second opinion that your Cousin Jack won't risk offending you with, or the news that the fund Uncle Howard wants you to buy is a dud.

MarketWatch.com has a masthead of about forty advisors like Merriman named the "RetireMentors," who contribute articles on all aspects of retirement finance. It's one of best resources available today.

> **FIVE WRONGS TO AVOID**
>
> Refusing to spend a little on an advisor is one of Paul Merriman's "5 Ways Most Investors Are Just Plain Wrong":
>
> - Blindly following pundits
> - Focusing on recent performance instead of long-term performance
> - Thinking mutual funds are risk-free
> - Believing fund sellers will protect you
> - Thinking advisors are a waste of money
>
> You can read the details at paulmerriman.com/5-ways-investors-just-plain-wrong/.

Retirement Coaches

If you have a ton of money to put into it, you can hire a retirement coach who will focus not on money and investments, but rather on finding your identity in retirement. The main idea is that you need to be prepared for the psychological transition from a high-powered career to a lower-key job or full retirement. One such coaching firm is NewDirections.com, (617) 523-7775, offering executive transition consulting. A lengthy report in *The New Yorker* points out that getting a "life portfolio" (that blends interests and aptitudes) is either a worthy goal or psycho-babble, depending on whether it works for you. You can find the article at Archives.NewYorker.com/?i=2012-10-08#folio=072.

Components of a Retirement Plan

Retirement planning can be as simple or as complicated as you want it to be. At the very least, you need to write down your expected income from all sources and your expected spending on all items and see where you stand.

If you are proficient with spreadsheets, you can make up your own retirement plan. If you are relatively financially literate, one of the best guides available today is Larry Swedroe's *The Only Guide You'll Ever Need for the Right Financial Plan*. If you are interested in managing your own finances, a good guide to get you up to speed is Paul Merriman's *Live It Up without Outliving Your Money*.

But if you are bored to tears or intimated into paralysis by finance, or just deeply uncomfortable with estimating future inflation and future rates of return, among other calculations and projections, this is reason enough to hire a retirement advisor. Before giving up entirely, howerver, to be able to evaluate what an advisor is telling you, you should take a crack at it yourself.

As in any financial undertaking, the plan has two parts — measuring what is coming in and measuring what is going out, to see how the two compare. If you have a monthly income of roughly $10,000 from a pension and Social Security, your current living costs are $5,000 (even before any downsizing), and if you also have a very large amount of savings, like $3 million, you don't need a retirement advisor — you need an investment advisor. But if your monthly income after retirement is $3,500 and your current expenses are $3500, with only $150,000 in savings, you need a retirement plan. You are not financially equipped to weather a single, large medical crisis or other big demand on your finances.

Measuring Outgo

Even if you never prepared a budget in your life, you really should start preparing one before you retire. People complain that they can't save a dime, but do not actually know in detail where their money is going. When it comes to money, the devil is in the details. You should collect all your bills, checks, and credit card statements, and do an honest accounting. In general, you will find expenses falling into fixed and variable categories — your mortgage is fixed; your telephone bill is variable.

Your spreadsheet should include these items:

- Rent or mortgage

- Home maintenance

- Utilities, including telephone

- Food

- Medical expenses, including prescription drugs

- Insurance: medical, life, auto, etc.

- Debt

- Taxes

- Clothing

- Pets, including medical costs

- Entertainment, including vacations

A FEW NOTES ON BUDGETS

- Acknowledge that your priorities will change. You may be happy to use only a cell phone and not to have a landline, but if you encounter health problems and live alone, you may want a hard-wired phone in every room.
- You may never have bought life insurance before, but unless you are wealthy, life insurance is an excellent remedy for survivors facing a loss of income.
- Be realistic about what you actually spend on food, pets, and entertainment.

The important thing is to project these expenses into the future at a rate of growth or a rate of inflation that will give you a realistic reading on your money needs. You should project out at least ten years, and then re-do the exercise every year. For example, you may be planning on downsizing your home — obviously you should use a new rent or mortgage amount. The cost of medical care until recently was rising faster than the overall rate of inflation. Data and information is available for overall inflation as well as specific items that make up the general indices at InflationData.com/inflation/Inflation_Articles/Calculate Inflation.asp.

The typical, US annual inflation rate is two percent (pre-retirement). You should use the forecast for inflation, increasing your expenses by two percent per year when you make your annual calculations. You don't have to become an expert on the economics of inflation, but it's smarter to use estimates from mainstream sources like the *Wall Street Journal* or EconoDay.com, than ideologically-influenced, scare-stories from the blogosphere.

Take a hard look at debt, too. Your goal should be to get and maintain a good credit score, even after you are retired. Credit card management advice from Clark Howard's *Living Large for the Long Haul* includes how to maintain a good credit score:

1. Always pay every bill on time (utilities, medical — everything).

2. Make a credit card payment every 14 days. Never let it get to a late fee.

3. Pay off the cards with the highest interest rate first.

4. Don't use more than 30 percent of your available credit (if total credit is $10,000, don't have a balance of more than $3,000).

5. Do not close credit card accounts! This only reduces your available credit and raises your usage rate.

   a. Instead, have four to six credit cards.

   b. Use each one twice a year and pay it down immediately. "Fifteen percent of your credit score is having open lines of credit that are responsibly managed."

6. Do not take store credit cards. They charge more interest and are not included in your credit score.

7. Get your credit bureau scores and dispute every single error. Consult AnnualCreditReport.com every four months (free). If credit bureaus do not fix errors, report it to the Consumer Financial Protection Bureau at ConsumerFinance.gov/complaint.

8. The most used score for auto and home loans is the FICO score from Equifax. Pay a fee at MyFico.com to get the FICO score ahead of time.

9. Never pay anyone to "repair" your credit. It can't be done and may worsen your rating.

10. If you negotiate with a credit card company to pay off a big amount with a lesser amount, get it in writing and be aware that the IRS will consider debt-forgiveness taxable income. This also lowers your rating.

11. As a near-last resort, consult the National Foundation for Credit Counseling, NFCC.org, (202) 677-4300 (free or low-cost).

12. Opt out of new credit card offerings at OptOutPrescreen.com.

13. To build credit, get a secured credit card (backed by a cash deposit) and ask the credit card company to convert it to a real credit card after 12–18 months. Some credit unions have a "fresh start" program.

Measuring Income

For most people, retirement income consists of a pension from an employer and Social Security. Unless you have a government pension, chances are you do not get any cost-of-living adjustments to your monthly benefit. Social Security benefits do receive a COLA adjustment every year, but as noted in Chapter 3, until recently the adjustment was insufficient to cover the true cost of medical care price increases that fall most heavily on the retired.

The other source of income is your savings and investments. These have two components: the base (capital) amount, and the rate of return. If you want to leave the principal amount untouched and take only the annual interest or dividends for regular expenses, you need to know the cash value of the return.

You can find rate of return calculators online, of which one of the best is at Bankrate.com. The easy-to-use calculator asks you to define some factors, like how many years you want to include in the analysis, your initial capital investment and any additions by year, your tax rate, and what kind of compounding you will be getting.

Simple interest pays a great deal less than compounding. Unfortunately, you also have to estimate some factors, including the rate of return you expect to get and the inflation rate (with

Bankrate conveniently including some standard benchmarks, like the 10-year-average rate of return on the S&P 500). In this calculation, the purpose of including an expected inflation rate is to increase contributions to the investment fund so that the total after-inflation amount is not eaten away by inflation. Bankrate offers many articles and examples on how to use the calculator, and even if you consider yourself an arithmetically-challenged, you can use it.

Putting Income and Outgo Together

Unless you are wealthy, chances are a realistic assessment of your projected financial condition will not be a cheerful prospect. You may have to reduce spending to increase savings and investments in order to have a rainy-day fund to draw on in case you need a new roof or a hip replacement. And one-time emergency use of your fund doesn't help with figuring out how much you can safely take out of capital every year for ordinary living expenses. A primitive methodology is to take the amount of total savings and investments and divide by your life expectancy. If you have another 25 years, according to the life expectancy tables, and you have $150,000 in savings (the US average), you can withdraw $5,000 per year, or $416.67 per month.

Be careful using a scheme like this. You could face a one-time catastrophic expense that would not just reduce, but use up the rest of your fund. You may also want to think of what will be left for survivors.

Don't forget the tax man. You are required to start withdrawing money from IRAs and other tax deferred investment accounts when you turn 70½. The IRS has been waiting for decades to collect those taxes! The "required minimum distribution" is described in gory detail at the IRS website and as noted in Chapter 1, the government uses your remaining life expectancy to calculate how much you must take out. And the IRS is heartless — if you take out less than you are required to take, the penalty is 50 percent of the difference between the minimum required and the actual amount you took (plus, of course, the taxes on the additional amount that tops up the withdrawal to the minimum).

The 4 Percent Rule

The old rule for withdrawing money from your rainy-day fund was that you could withdraw four percent per year, and then four percent plus the actual rate of inflation every year thereafter and not run out of money for three decades.

The *4 percent rule* was devised by financial planners who were basing it on the historical returns on a conventional portfolio consisting of 60 percent equities/40 percent bonds. In the early 1990s, the set of 30-year spans starting with 1926–1955 would have generated the right amount of return to allow a four percent withdrawal rate. The problem, of course, is that in 2008 we had a 38 percent drop in the S&P, and as described in Chapter 7, when you began investing is really important. According to broker T. Rowe Price, "If you had retired January 1, 2000, with an initial four percent withdrawal rate and a portfolio of 55 percent stocks and 45 percent bonds rebalanced each month, with the first year's withdrawal amount increased by three percent per year for inflation, your portfolio would have fallen by a third through 2010 . . . And you would be left with only a 29 percent chance of making it through three decades."

Don't put your head in the sand when it comes to the financial aspect of retirement. Taken step by step, financial planning doesn't have to be a scary prospect. The following advice will put you on the road to making a solid retirement plan:

DaVINCI DO'S

- Equip yourself to interview planners by doing some research and have your base plan already in hand.

- Paul Merriman offers sound investment advice. Read his columns online or perhaps pick up one of his books.

- Be aware of potential frauds and scams. Sign up for the AARP's Fraud Watch Network at AARP.org/money/scams-fraud/fraud-watch-network, and check the FBI's website for the latest scams and frauds at FBI.gov/scams-safety/fraud/seniors.

DaVINCI DON'TS

- Don't allow late planning or slim savings to shame you out of getting the investment advice that you need.

- When creating a budgetary forecast, don't forget to increase your expenses by at least three percent per year to account for inflation.

- Be careful and wary of retirement planners and investment advisors, but not so fearful that you fail to consult any planner, or worse, fail to attempt a financial retirement plan yourself. And again, when you find a planner with whom you're comfortable, don't be afraid to spend a bit of money for financial advisement.

Health Considerations

The Long and Winding Road to Long-Term Care

9

SEVEN IN 10. That's how many Americans 65 and older will one day require some form of long-term care in a residential facility, nursing home, adult day-care center, or in their own homes, according to the US Department of Health and Human Services.

One in 12. The number of Americans who have actually purchased long-term insurance to pay for it, according to the October 2013 Harris Interactive/HealthDay survey.

If you don't think those twin statistics add up to a significant problem for the nation's legion of aging baby boomers, consider the following facts and figures:

- The fastest-growing segment of the US population is seniors over 85 years of age, according to the US Census Bureau. But while medical advances are allowing Americans to live longer than ever before, health statistics show a growing number of

US seniors are also living with chronic health conditions that make them more likely to require long-term care.

- Nearly half the population — 46 percent — of people 85 and older will develop Alzheimer's or dementia requiring assisted medical and/or residential care, according to the Alzheimer's Association. In many cases, adult children live in separate cities and are unable to help out with their parents' needs.

- Nearly 12 million Americans now require some form of long-term care, according to the US Department of Health and Human Services — 37 percent of whom were under age 65. That number is expected to skyrocket as the US population ages.

- More than two-thirds of Americans (68 percent) say they are uncertain about how they'll meet long-term care costs should they need them, the Harris poll suggests. Most people don't know how such costs are now covered, with about half mistakenly believing bills are primarily paid by individuals, one-third falsely thinking Medicare pays, and 81 percent not realizing the main funder of long-term care is Medicaid, which covers health services for the poor.

The one thing most people get right is that the situation is reaching crisis proportions, with 87 percent surveyed in the Harris poll saying the problem of how to pay for seniors' long-term care will only get worse as the nation ages, calling the situation "serious" or "somewhat serious."

Translation: Many Americans are unprepared for the future and may be forced to turn to the only option available — Medicaid, the nation's healthcare program for the poor — to pay the costs of their care.

But it doesn't have to be this way. You can — and should — buy private insurance that specifically covers long-term care. While it can be pricey, particularly for those over the age of 60, the Harris poll found nearly two-thirds of Americans think "most people" would benefit from long-term care insurance; health and financial experts agree. There are other steps you can also take to prepare and plan ahead.

Of course, it would help if the government provided bigger tax breaks to help people purchase long-term care insurance. But the sweeping Patient Protection and Affordable Care Act of 2010 (also known as ObamaCare) does nothing to address the issue and there are no firm plans on the table for other programs to create such financial incentives.

The authors of ObamaCare initially sought to address the nation's long-term care crisis, but those plans have been shelved. Tucked into the 2,500-plus pages of ObamaCare is a little-known provision designed to provide financial help for the long-term care of those who need assistance with basic living tasks made difficult with age or disability. But the so-called CLASS provision — short for "Community Living Assistance and Supports" — proved to be very controversial, largely because regulations required enrollee contributions to entirely pay for its operations before it could get up and running. In October 2011, the White House officially suspended the CLASS program over concerns that enrollment levels would be very low (participation was voluntary) and that taxpayers would end up funding another massive health-related entitlement program.

One reason federal officials sought to create the CLASS program in the first place is that many of the nation's major insurers no longer offer new long-term care policies. In fact, *Consumer Reports* magazine recently stated that over past five years, 10 of the top 20 insurers (by sales) have stopped selling new, long-term-care plans to individuals, according to LIMRA International, an insurance industry research company.

At the same time, premiums are rising for those who already hold such policies. A policy purchased in 2012 cost as much as 17 percent more than a year earlier, based on the latest projections from the American Association for Long-Term Care Insurance, an industry group. The reason: Insurers overestimated how many people would stop paying for their policies over time and underestimated the costs of such care.

7 Key Questions and Answers to Long-Term Care

In light of these political and economic realities, you must take proactive steps to plan for the future by taking the time to understand the various types of long-term care; the assistance state and federal agencies provide (and don't); planning for the cost of such care (which may include purchasing an insurance policy for coverage before age 60, at which point premiums soar); understanding tax breaks for premiums and benefit payments; and creating a plan for your future, perhaps with the help of a professional.

The answers to the following seven questions will help you get started:

No. 1: What Is Long-Term Care?

Unlike other forms of healthcare, long-term care provides help with basic tasks involved with day-to-day living for people who can't manage them on their own. It can include a range of options:

Home healthcare typically involves an aide, nurse, and/or therapist who comes to the home to provide a few hours of help each day or a few times a week. That may include assistance with meals, bathing, dressing, using the bathroom, getting into/out of bed, and other basic tasks of living. Other common services and supports include help with housework, managing money, taking medication, shopping for groceries or clothes, using the phone or other communication devices, and caring for pets.

Adult day care programs allow for older adults to spend a morning or afternoon (or both) at a center with trained professionals. Some also provide transportation to and from the home.

Assisted living or nursing home facilities provide round-the-clock residential and medical care, including the provision of meals, recreation, entertainment, and medication, along with help bathing, dressing, and managing other daily needs.

Hospice care involves end-of-life services, either in a resident's home or a hospice facility.

For individuals without a spouse or adult child who can be a full-time, primary caregiver, at least some outside help is usually required, depending on the level of physical or mental disability.

No. 2: Is Such Care Pricey?

In a word: Yes. According to a 2013 analysis of long-term care policies by *Consumer Reports* magazine:

- A private room in a highly-rated, skilled nursing home can cost as much as $10,000 per month (with the national average hovering just over a staggering $6,200).

- A single-bedroom unit in an assisted-living facility averages about half of that monthly cost — about $3,200 — but is still expensive.

- Adult day care centers typically fetch between $60 and $70 per day.

- Standard fees for home healthcare aides vary widely by state, but are typically the lowest-cost option — averaging just over $20 per hour, depending on the services provided.

No. 3: How Much Do Long-Term Insurance Policies Cost?

Like other kinds of insurance policies, costs for long-term plans vary widely by state, region, facility, age, health status, and coverage and benefit levels. But most pick up at least some expenses related to home healthcare, hospice care, adult day care, and stays in a nursing home or assisted-living facility.

Like other forms of insurance, you'll pay less for coverage if you purchase a plan when you are younger and healthier than if you wait until you are over the age of 60 and/or have a chronic health condition.

According to the National Association of Insurance Commissioners, if you buy a new, long-term care insurance policy when you hit 50, you can expect to pay an average of about $900 a year if you are generally in good health. If you wait until you're 65, you'll pay more than twice as much — close to $1,850. And if you don't buy a plan until you're 75, you'll have to pony up about $6,000 per year.

Unlike traditional health insurance, long-term policies cover services and supports, including personal and custodial care in a variety of settings such as, your home, a community organization, or other facility. They typically reimburse policyholders a daily amount (up to a pre-selected limit) for services to assist them with activities of daily living (bathing, dressing, eating, etc.). You can select a range of care

MAINTAINING RATES

For most long-term care policies, you need to keep paying your premiums to maintain your rates — which are calculated based on the date you first take out such a plan. If you stop making payments, most policies automatically terminate and you'll lose any benefits you've accrued. Some policies will allow you to preserve some benefits if you stop paying, but only after you've held the policy for a period of years and agree to pay higher premiums once you resume payments.

options and benefits that allow you to get the services you need, where you need them.

The cost of your policy is based on:

- Your age

- The maximum amount the policy will pay per day

- The number of days (years) it will pay (the lifetime maximum is based on the amount of coverage per day multiplied by the number of days it will be in effect)

- Any optional benefits you choose

If you are in poor health, you may not qualify for insurance or will have to buy a more limited amount of coverage at a higher rate. Be sure to determine ahead of time if any policy you wish to buy will cover you for a set period of years (often two to five) or for as long as you live. You should also know an insurance company may raise the premium on your policy, so it's wise to review a company's past history on premium rate hikes.

No. 4: Is Insurance the Only Option?

No. Many people think the phrase "long-term care" is synonymous with insurance, but buying such a policy is only one way to prepare for such care and may only be one part of your plan. A number of other options can help cover long-term care, including reverse mortgages, annuities, and life insurance policies.

A reverse mortgage, as discussed in Chapter 4, is a home equity loan that essentially pays you cash against the value of your home without requiring you to sell it or move out of it. In most cases you can choose to receive a monthly payment, a single lump-sum payment, or a line of credit. Because there are no restrictions on how you use that money — you are free to purchase long-term care with it. Most people continue to reside in the home, retain title and ownership, and are still responsible for property insurance, home maintenance, and taxes. With a reverse mortgage, you do not need to repay the loan as long as you live in the home, but the amount you owe — based on loan payouts and interest — is due when you or the last borrower, such as a spouse, dies, sells, or moves out. To qualify, you must be at least 62 years of age.

An annuity contract with an insurance company can help you pay for long-term care. In exchange for a single payment or a series of payments, an insurer will send you an annuity — a series of regular payments for a set period of time. With an "immediate annuity" you receive a specific monthly income in return for a single premium payment, regardless of your health status (which makes such a policy attractive to anyone in poor health). How much you receive depends on the amount of your initial premium, your age, and gender. With a "deferred annuity" an insurer creates two funds — one for long-term care expenses and a second for you to use however you wish. Such plans are available to people up to age 85 and allow you to access the long-term care funds immediately, but you must wait until a preset time in the future to access the cash portion.

ANNUITY TAX EFFECT

The effect that annuities can have on your taxes is complicated, so it's a good idea to consult a tax attorney or accountant before purchasing one.

Life insurance policies can also be used to pay for long-term care through the following options:

- **Combination life/long-term care insurance products** allow consumers to combine both types of policies, which guarantee that policy benefits will always be paid, in one form or another. These products are relatively new, but the amount of the long-term benefit is usually a percentage of the life insurance benefit.

- **Accelerated death benefits** (ADBs) can be included in some life insurance policies that allow you to receive a tax-free advance on your benefit before you die, often by paying a higher premium. Depending on the type of ADB policy you have, you may be able to receive a cash advance on your life insurance policy's death benefit if you become terminally ill or require long-term care at home or in a nursing facility. For most policies that cover long-term care, the monthly benefit is usually about two percent of the life insurance policy's face value (and more limited than what you'd receive from a typical long-term plan). An average example is provided by HHS: If your life insurance policy's face value is $200,000, then the monthly payout available to you for care in a nursing home would be $4,000, but only $2,000 for home care. Any

TABLE 9-1: LIFE EXPECTANCY VS. BENEFITS	
Life Expectancy	Benefit (by percentage)
1-6 months	80%
6-12 months	70%
12-18 months	65%
18-25 months	60%
Over 24 months	50%

Source: The US Department of Health and Human Services,
http://longtermcare.gov/costs-how-to-pay/using-life-insurance-to-pay-for-long-term-care/

The cash you receive from a viatical settlement is a percentage of the death benefit on your life insurance policy, and that percent varies based on your life expectancy.

payments made for long-term care are then subtracted from the amount paid to your beneficiaries when you die.

- **Life settlements** are plans that allow you to sell your life insurance policy to raise cash for long-term care, or other reasons. This option is usually only available to women aged 74 and older and to men aged 70 and older, and the proceeds of the sale are subject to taxes.

- **Viatical settlements** are similar to life settlements, in that they allow you to sell your life insurance policy to a third party and use the money you receive to pay for long-term care, but they can only be used if you are terminally ill and have a life expectance of two years or less. A viatical company pays you a percentage of the death benefit on your life insurance policy, based on your life expectancy, and becomes the owner and beneficiary when you die in exchange for taking over payment of the premiums on the policy. Unlike the life settlement, money you receive from a viatical settlement is tax-free.

No. 5: Won't Medicare Pay for Some Long-Term Care?

Yes and no. In some cases, Medicare will pay for several months' stay in a skilled nursing home or assisted-living facility, but only after an illness, injury, or hospitalization.

In general, Medicare only pays for long-term care if you require skilled services or rehabilitative care in a nursing home for a maximum of 100 days (the average Medicare-covered stay is just 22 days). Medicare will also cover some in-home services if you are also receiving skilled home health or other skilled in-home services, but only for a short time. But Medicare won't cover costs of an aide providing assistance with most daily-living tasks.

For these reasons, it's best not to bank on Medicare to provide for any extended stay you may need in a residential-care facility.

No. 6: What about Medicaid?

Medicaid, the federal health program for the nation's poor and disabled, pays for the largest share of long-term care services in the nation. But to qualify for Medicaid, your monthly income must be less than the federal poverty level, and your assets cannot exceed certain limits. Such requirements are based on the amount of assistance you need with daily-living tasks.

Also, Medicaid will cover you only in nursing homes and in certain home healthcare arrangements that offer the level of care you need.

States have different standards for Medicaid eligibility. Most use the same asset and income-limit guidelines set by the federal Supplemental Security Income program (SSI), but some have their own income and asset guidelines. In real terms, residents of most states can make up to 300 percent of the SSI income limit ($2,163 per month, based on 2014 rates) and still qualify for nursing-home-only Medicaid. Most states also allow those who meet these guidelines but are "medically needy" to qualify for Medicaid.

For the states that use the SSI standards, there is a $2,000 limit on countable assets for one person ($3,000 per married couple). But SSI/Medicaid does not count all resources. For example, primary residences are usually not counted (up to a certain amount of equity, depending on your home state).

If you have assets that put you over the Medicaid limit, you must "spend down" your resources below the limit or pay out-of-pocket to enter a nursing home or assisted living facility, until your assets meet the eligibility guidelines. Some individuals give their resources and assets away to qualify for Medicaid, but there are limits to such gifts (i.e., you can't give a second home to your children). In addition, Medicaid officials will look back five years to see whether you gave away anything for less than fair market value during that time, which would disqualify you for coverage.

Some states have programs designed to help people with the financial impact of spending down to meet Medicaid eligibility standards. Under these programs, you buy a federally qualified partnership policy to become eligible. For more information, check with your state insurance department or a counseling program.

Other federal programs, such as the Older Americans Act and the Department of Veterans Affairs, pay for long-term care services, but only for specific populations and in certain circumstances.

No 7: How Can You Tell if You're Likely to Need Long-Term Care?

Federal statistics show some people are more likely to require at least some long-term care as they age. Among them:

- Women, who outlive men by about five years on average, are more likely to live at home and require assistance in their later years.

- Being involved in an accident or suffering from a chronic illness, such as diabetes, high blood pressure, or any physical impairment or illness that causes a disability increases the likelihood you'll need care. If your parents or grandparents had chronic conditions, that may increase your odds of requiring long-term care. Poor diet and exercise habits boost your chances of needing long-term care.

- Advancing age is the biggest factor. About 69 percent of people aged 90 or above have a disability requiring long-term care. Eight percent of Americans between 40 and 50 have a disability that could require assistance. Someone turning age 65 today has a 70 percent chance of needing some type of long-term care; 20 percent of those individuals will need it for longer than five years.

- More people use long-term care services at home (and for longer) than in facilities. Such care is often provided by family members or friends, with about 67 million Americans — one in four — cared for by unpaid caregivers, who provide at least 20 hours of services a week.

Finally, these basic guidelines should be used as an initial yardstick when considering or shopping for long-term care:

DaVINCI DO'S

- Evaluate the likelihood you will need some form of long-term care before age 60, at which point insurance costs rise dramatically. About 70 percent of Americans will need such care, but only one in 12 actually purchases insurance to pay for it.

- Compare and contrast the types of care that would be suitable to you. Home healthcare aides, nurses, or therapists provide a few hours of help each day or a few times a week, while adult day care programs allow older adults to spend a morning or afternoon (or both) at a center with trained professionals. Assisted living or nursing homes provide round-the-clock residential and medical care, including meals, recreation, help bathing, dressing, and managing other daily needs.

- Check with your state's Center for Independent Living for detailed assistance and resources on long-term care and facilities for people with disabilities of all ages and incomes. A state-by-state listing of CILs can be found at the center's website at: NCIL.org, or call (202) 207-0334.

DaVINCI DON'TS

- Never choose a nursing home or long-term care facility for a loved one without checking the home's record and inspection history by visiting your home state's Medicaid or insurance division website. You can also check the federal Medicare website for background information at Medicare.gov/nursinghome compare/search.html?AspxAutoDetectCookieSupport=1.

- Don't presume your Medicare plan will cover you should you need long-term care. The US Department of Health and Human Services website details the limitations of coverage within Medicare and provides other resources on long-term care at LongTermCare.gov/the-basics.

- If you're a caregiver providing assistance to a disabled spouse, relative, or friend, don't try to go it alone. The Family Caregiver Alliance is an advocacy group that offers advice and support for caregivers through its website Caregiver.org.

The Silver Tsunami

IT IS THE LARGEST demographic wave in our nation's history: Over the next two decades, the number of Americans turning 65 will double — topping more than 75 million by the year 2030. That's about 10,000 people per day — every day — between now and 2029.

The impact of this "Silver Tsunami" is likely to fundamentally change who we are and how we live — impacting our politics, economy, retirement lifestyles, consumer habits, culture, and even the way we think about what it means to be old.

But nowhere will those effects be felt as strongly as in the field of healthcare, impacting Medicare, the nation's program for elderly and disabled residents. Many experts believe Medicare as we know it today is likely to be swamped by the rising wave of eligible baby boomers unless major structural and financial changes are made to make sure it remains solvent.

Consider the following:

- When Medicare was created in 1965, 19 million Americans were eligible. Today, it's more than 50 million — 10 million more than just a decade ago — and that figure is rising by the day, according to federal Centers for Medicare & Medicaid Services (CMS).

- In 2010, the federal government spent $528 billion to support the program. By 2020, that spending is projected to hit $1 trillion.

- When Medicare first went into effect, the monthly premium for Part B (medical insurance) was only $3. By 2010, Part A (hospital premium) cost up to $461 per person per month, and Part B cost more than $96 per individual.

- Average benefits for recipients today: Almost $12,100 (with average medical costs around $15,000), according to the nonpartisan Kaiser Family Foundation.

- Average life expectancy when Medicare was created 50 years ago: 70. Today: nearly 80 years of age.

- A woman turning 65 today can expect to live until age 86, on average, which is two years longer than the average life expectancy of a 65-year-old man, according to the Social Security Administration. About one in every four 65-year-olds today will live past age 90.

Few would argue Medicare's success. Prior to 1965, about half of American seniors had no health insurance whatsoever, and many others had poor coverage, at best. But the advent of Medicare guaranteed that seniors would have health plans comparable to high-quality, employer-sponsored insurance.

Many health experts also believe the program has contributed to the rapid rise in life expectancy in the United States, while also reducing the poverty rate for American seniors, which has fallen by 50 percent over the past half-century, according to the National Bipartisan Commission on the Future of Medicare.

But Medicare is facing serious financial and health-related challenges. Over the next 30 years, as the number of beneficiaries doubles, the ratio of Medicare recipients to workers — whose taxes fund more than half of program — is projected to fall from

1:4 to about 2:1. As a result, the nonpartisan Congressional Budget Office predicts that the program will be bankrupt without significant changes in eligibility guidelines, covered services, and financing.

In fact, changes in federal funding for Medicare included in the $85 billion in cuts mandated by the Budget Control Act in 2013 — the sequester — spotlight trims that seniors should be concerned about in the years ahead. Among them:

- **Hospitals**: Decreases in Medicare reimbursement for the nation's 3,500 hospitals and skilled nursing facilities totaled nearly $4.5 billion — or about $1.3 million for the average facility — resulting in many layoffs, especially nurses ($1.3 million is equivalent to 25 full-time positions).

- **Physicians:** Medicare payments to doctors dropped by two percent, totaling $4.1 billion. Over the past decade Medicare payments for physician services have inched up by four percent, while the cost of caring for patients has soared by 20 percent. That mandated two percent cut only widened this gap and adds to pressures that may push physicians to stop accepting Medicare patients or decide to retire early, contributing to already-serious doctor shortages in many areas of the country in the years ahead.

The Politics of Medicare

The debate over ObamaCare has also turned Medicare into a political football. During the 2012 presidential campaign, for instance, Democrats and Republicans each accused the other side of seeking to "cut or gut" the federal government's health insurance program for seniors and the disabled.

But, politics aside, the fiery campaign rhetoric neatly framed the coming debate on Medicare, offering a glimpse of the ways Washington is likely to modify and alter the federal program over the next decade , having a significant impact on seniors.

Mitt Romney accused President Barack Obama of "cutting" Medicare, which GOP campaign officials have charged could lead to benefit limits and the rationing of healthcare for seniors. The president and his operatives argued, however, that the administration's plans and proposals have only strengthened Medicare and produced tangible benefits for seniors.

But the truth is that the leaders of both political parties in Congress have proposed plans that seek to limit the growth in spending for the program. Technically, those reductions aren't "cuts" to the existing Medicare budget (although it is an accepted term to describe budgetary spending reductions), but rather limits on spending increases over time.

Why does the federal government need to hold down Medicare costs? As former president Bill Clinton and Republican Florida Sen. Marco Rubio have both rightly noted, it's not politics, it's math.

As more of the nation's baby boomers turn 65 and fewer younger working Americans are left to pay into the program, without a fix, Medicare is heading for disaster. The number of people enrolled in Medicare will grow to roughly 80 million when the last of the baby boomers turns 65 in two decades, according to the nonprofit Pew Research Center. Without action, that would nearly double the amount spent each year on the program from about $500 billion to $1 trillion.

To ratchet down those costs, the Obama administration — in provisions contained in the Patient Protection and Affordable Care Act (ObamaCare) — proposes to trim $716 billion in Medicare spending through the year 2022, according to the nonpartisan Congressional Budget Office.

Romney's vice-presidential running mate, US Rep. Paul Ryan, included the same amount of Medicare spending reductions in his own budget proposals as chairman of the House Budget Committee. Most of those proposed reductions are for reimbursements to hospitals and insurers.

Both sides maintain that their own budget plans will largely leave Medicare unchanged for Americans today.

The Obama administration says the trims will have no significant negative impacts on seniors' Medicare benefits, adding that additional provisions of ObamaCare have given seniors assistance in closing the so-called "donut hole" in prescription drug coverage. The new law also pays for yearly, no-cost wellness visits and preventive services, such as cancer screenings, diabetes tests, and flu shots.

But the law also requires higher-income Medicare beneficiaries to pay more for drug coverage. Medicare beneficiaries who earn more than $85,000 ($170,000 for a couple) now pay higher premiums for drugs, as well as physician and outpatient services, under ObamaCare.

In addition, many experts note that cutting $716 billion from any government program is sure to have downstream impacts on benefits and costs to seniors; some even argue ObamaCare's provisions could lead to rationing and other negative healthcare effects.

One other way ObamaCare seeks to keep Medicare solvent is to raise taxes paid by higher-income Americans for hospital-related insurance expenditures for the nation's seniors. As of January 1, 2013, Medicare taxes rose to 3.8 percent — from 2.9 percent the year before — for taxpayers who earn more than $200,000 a year and married couples earning $250,000 filing jointly.

The IPAB: "Death Panel" or Expert Board of Directors?

A more controversial bone of contention concerns the Affordable Care Act's provision to create a presidential commission called the Independent Payment Advisory Board (IPAB). This board of 15 experts — chosen by the president and approved by the Senate — would have the power to force additional Medicare cuts if costs rise beyond certain levels and Congress fails to act. Its decisions could only be counteracted by a three-fifths "super-majority" vote in Congress.

The driving idea behind the IPAB's creation is that the board would be able to make tough budgetary decisions that might be politically difficult for Congress or the president to implement (such as additional Medicare reductions). But because the IPAB won't be elected, critics argue the board could wield enormous powers and increase government control over the Medicare system.

During the 2012 presidential debates with Obama, Romney referred to the IPAB as "an unelected board that's going to tell people ultimately what kind of treatments they can have. I don't like that idea." His comments echoed assertions made by many critics that Obama's law would lead to rationing, made famous by former Alaska Gov. Sarah Palin's widely debunked allegation that it would create "death panels."

But Obama administration officials note the healthcare law explicitly prohibits the board from rationing care, shifting costs to retirees, restricting benefits, or raising the Medicare eligibility age. So the board doesn't have the power to dictate to doctors what treatments they can prescribe.

"Premium Support" Payments: Voucher Program?

While both sides insist their plans will leave Medicare's administration largely unchanged for now, the Republicans and Democrats have very different ideas about how to preserve the program down the road, beginning in 2022.

Obama and fellow Democrats say the best way to keep Medicare solvent is to leave the entitlement program intact, but strengthen its ability to pay for quality.

Romney and others have proposed converting Medicare from a guaranteed benefit program to a system providing fixed "premium support" payments that beneficiaries could use to purchase coverage either from traditional Medicare or a private insurer, based on a sliding scale tied to income.

Democratic critics deride the GOP plan as a "voucher" system, which Republicans say is misleading. But unanswered questions remain for both plans.

Critics of ObamaCare argue that Democratic leaders have not detailed how Medicare could hope to keep the program solvent while covering the exploding number of seniors who will qualify for the program by 2022, given significantly reduced revenues from working Americans.

Critics of Romney's "premium support" plan contend GOP leaders have not made clear how or even whether it would guarantee essential health services for seniors. They also argue it could leave beneficiaries vulnerable in coming years to rising, out-of-pocket healthcare costs, including private insurance premiums, and endanger traditional Medicare by leaving it to care for only the sickest people.

One thing seems all but certain: Retirees are likely to shoulder an increasing percentage of costs under Medicare over time, regardless of how the plan changes.

Coming up With a Medicare Game Plan

So what does this all mean for you? If you're currently receiving Medicare or are approaching the age of eligibility, you already know how daunting a task it can be to pick a plan. In many states with large senior populations, such as California and Florida, dozens — or even hundreds — of choices are available, making the job of selecting the right plan nearly as difficult as buying a new car or house.

You need to evaluate not only costs and prices, but also whether your doctors are part of the plan, what prescription medicines are paid for (and not), and what extra benefits are covered, such as eye exams, dental care, wellness visits, and even "Silver Sneakers" health club memberships.

So where do you start? Here are fifteen questions (and answers) to help you plan, prepare, and pick a health plan. Be aware, there is no one-size-fits-all solution; your choice should be based on your individual needs. You should also know that numerous national and state-based advocacy groups (listed at the end of this chapter) can help you choose a suitable plan and navigate the difficult changes in Medicare that are likely to take place in the coming decade, and beyond.

But the following questions will at least get you thinking about priorities and provide some textbook examples that will help you do your homework. Good luck!

NO. 1: WHO IS COVERED BY MEDICARE?

Medicare insurance is for:

- Seniors 65 or older.

- Some Americans under 65 with certain disabilities.

- Anyone with end-stage renal disease, permanent kidney failure requiring dialysis or an organ transplant, or amyotrophic lateral sclerosis (ALS, also known as Lou Gehrig's disease).

In general, if you qualify for Social Security you are also eligible for Medicare. You must be a legal US citizen and you (or your spouse) must have worked and paid payroll taxes for at least 10 years. If you don't quality under these rules, you may still be able to gain some Medicare coverage by paying a monthly fee.

NO. 2: WHAT ARE THE PRIMARY ELEMENTS OF MEDICARE?

Medicare covers basic medical services (like lab tests, surgeries, and doctor visits) and "medically necessary" supplies (like wheelchairs and walkers) required to treat a health condition. It also covers preventive healthcare services and prescription drugs. If you're in a Medicare Advantage Plan or other specialized Medicare plans, you may have to live by certain rules and face limits on some services.

But, in general, Medicare is divided in four major components:

1. Medicare Part A

Covers in-patient care in hospitals, temporary nursing home stays, hospice, as well as home health services.

2. Medicare Part B

Covers services or tests you get from your doctor in his or her office, a hospital, outpatient facility, a skilled nursing facility, your home or other settings, mental health, medical equipment, lab services, diagnostic tests, and ambulance service. Such services are required to diagnose or treat your medical condition and must meet accepted standards of medical practice. A doctor can be a medical doctor (MD), a doctor of osteopathy (DO), or, in some cases, a specialist, such as a dentist, podiatrist, optometrist, chiropractor, physician assistant, nurse practitioner, clinical nurse specialist, clinical social worker, physical and occupational therapist, speech/language pathologist, or clinical psychologist.

ALSO KNOWN AS

Parts A and B are sometimes called "traditional Medicare."

Part B also covers ambulance services, durable medical equipment, mental healthcare — including in-patient, outpatient, and in-hospital treatment — and some outpatient prescription drugs. It generally covers 80 percent of Medicare-approved coverage for services, after your deductible has been met. In addition, Part B covers 100 percent of preventive healthcare services designed to ward off illness (like the flu) or detect it at an early stage (cancer, diabetes, heart disease), when treatment is most likely to work best.

3. Medicare Part C

Also known as Medicare Advantage Plans, Part C are alternative health plans offered by private companies that contract with Medicare to provide all Part A and Part B benefits, and usually other aspects of care, such as prescription drug coverage (Medicare Part D), vision plans, and dental care — sometimes for an extra fee. (Medicare Advantage Plans with prescription drug coverage are sometimes called "MA-PDs." Medicare Advantage Plans include Health Maintenance Organizations, Preferred Provider Organizations, Private Fee-for-Service Plans, Special Needs Plans, and Medicare Medical Savings Account Plans.)

4. Medicare Part D

These Prescription Drug Plans are free-standing programs run by private Medicare-approved insurers to provide drug coverage. These plans (sometimes called "PDPs") add drug coverage to a traditional Medicare plan (which does not contain coverage for medicines), as well as some Medicare Cost Plans, Medicare Private Fee-for-Service (PFFS) Plans, and Medicare Medical Savings Account (MSA) Plans. Drug-only plans may also be good options if you have medical coverage from a private insurer, an employer, or another federal agency that doesn't cover prescription drugs. They are for individuals who do not have a Medicare Advantage Plan (Part C) or other Medicare health plan that offers Medicare prescription drug coverage. Choosing a Part D plan can help lower the cost of prescription drugs and protect you from higher costs in the future. When you join a Medicare drug plan, you'll give your Medicare number and the date your Part A and/or Part B coverage started.

> **BEWARE: AUTO RENEW**
>
> Medicare Advantage and prescription drug plans will automatically renew for the next year unless you take steps to opt out. It's always a good idea to comparison shop, even if you think you have the best Part C and D plans, because they change year-to-year and you may find your doctors, hospitals, or drug coverage may change, as well as monthly premiums, deductibles, and co-pays.

Other Medicare Health Plans

Some other types of Medicare health plans provide Part A and/or Part B coverage, as well as prescription drug coverage, that follow the same rules as Medicare Advantage Plans. Examples include Medicare Cost Plans and Programs of All-inclusive Care for the Elderly (PACE).

In addition, seniors can choose to buy "Medigap" supplement policies — private plans that cover out-of-pocket expenses not covered by their policies, including deductibles, co-payments, and other costs.

Medicare also runs a series of demonstrations or pilot programs that are special projects designed to test improvements in

Medicare coverage, payment, and healthcare quality. They usually operate only for a limited time for a specific group of people and/or are offered only in specific areas.

For instance, Medicare officials are experimenting with so-called Accountable Care Organizations — ACOs — that aim to build teams of doctors, including general practitioners and specialists working together in efficient, coordinated harmony to collaboratively plan and carry out patient care and be paid in "bundled payments." The ultimate goal is to use them to replace the current fee-for-service system with ACOs. ObamaCare creates a new demonstration project that allows ACOs with at least 5,000 Medicare recipients to participate. Each ACO that signs up must accept all patients, even those in the worst health. The program works like this:

- **Hospitals, physicians and home-care providers** work together to deliver comprehensive and continuous care to each patient who agrees to participate.

- **Each member of the treatment team is paid** on a fee-for-service basis.

- **Bonuses are paid out** for quality care that is delivered below a given dollar threshold (to be determined by the Department of Health and Human Services).

The program began in January 2012 and is slated to last three years. ACO cost savings are expected to be five to 10 percent.

So far, more than 250 individual Medicare ACOs have been approved by the White House and are in operation, serving about four million of the nation's 50 million Medicare patients. They are expected to save as much as $5-10 billion over the next eight years.

If you're interested in checking out a demonstration or pilot program to see if it might work for you, call (800) MEDICARE , or (800) 633-4227.

NO. 3: DO YOU EVEN NEED MEDICARE?

The truth is that many seniors don't even need to become Medicare beneficiaries. If you already have retiree health benefits from a previous job, a current employer, spousal insurance, or a Veterans

Affairs plan, your coverage may be equal to — or better than — what a traditional Medicare plan can offer.

Alternatively, you may want to boost your coverage with a supplement plan or a Medicare Advantage policy that will give you greater coverage for prescription drugs, doctor visits, and other care.

NO. 4: SHOULD YOU STICK WITH YOUR CURRENT MEDICARE PLAN?

If you currently have a Medicare plan that you like, you may want to simply re-up your coverage-stay with that insurer. But before making that decision to lock in, be sure to check what's called a "Notice of Change," supplied by your insurer, for any alterations in costs, premiums, coverage levels, and other benefits for the next year.

Plans typically change year-to year. So it's also a good idea to at least shop around and see what's offered by other plans, for comparison. You may be able to get a better deal by making a switch, but you won't know if you don't do an apples-to-apples comparison.

NO. 5: WHAT TYPE OF PLAN WORKS BEST FOR YOU AND YOUR BUDGET?

Medicare plans typically come in three varieties — pricey, private fee-for-service (PFFS) plans, mid-priced preferred provider organizations (PPOs), and bargain-basement health maintenance organizations (HMOs). Each type of plan has its own advantages and disadvantages — with varying costs, coverage levels, and limitations.

PFFS give you the greatest freedom to choose doctors and healthcare facilities, without a referral from a primary care doctor. They also typically provide the most generous coverage levels. But the downside is that they are generally the costliest plans available.

PPOs are next in line in terms of cost and coverage levels, carrying lower premiums than PFFs and covering at least some out-of-network care (often for a higher, but not prohibitively expensive cost) without a referral. Most also offer prescription drug plans that typically favor generic medications.

HMOs have the lowest premiums of all plans, but restrict you to a limited network of physicians and hospitals. They also require referrals for you to see a specialist, which can sometimes be cumbersome and take time to work out with insurers. They typically carry drug plans, but may limit what types of brand-name medicines they will cover.

But whichever type of plan you choose, make sure your regular doctors, preferred healthcare facilities, and prescription medications are covered before you enroll.

NO. 6: DO YOU QUALIFY FOR A DISCOUNT?

If you are on a limited income and have few assets, it's possible you could qualify for help with all or part of your Medicare premiums, deductibles, co-payments, or prescription drug costs. As of 2014, individuals with incomes under $17,505 and assets less than $13,440, and couples with incomes under $23,595 and assets less than $26,860 qualify for subsidies. People who have chronic health conditions, such as heart disease, cancer, and diabetes, or live in nursing homes may also qualify for special needs assistance.

For more information, contact Social Security at (800) 772-1213 or go to SocialSecurity.gov.

NO. 7: WHEN CAN YOU SIGN UP?

The enrollment typically runs from mid-October through early December each year to secure coverage for the following year that begins January 1. If you miss the enrollment deadline, you may have to stick with the plan you have until the following fall.

Consumer advocates recommend comparing plans year to year, even if you decide you want to keep your plan. Most have at least some subtle changes, so doing a comparison of plans offered each year will help guarantee you are making the best choice possible. You should also make sure your needs haven't changed — new medications, the need for specialists, or other factors that may require a change in your health plan.

It's also a good idea to check your plan's network of covered providers, drug stores, and healthcare facilities each year, since those can change as well. Many doctors are no longer offering Medicare services because of federal changes in the law and reimbursement rates that have not risen to keep pace with the cost of caring for Medicare patients.

For all these reasons, it's important to evaluate your Medicare plan year-to-year and adjust as needed.

NO. 8: ARE THERE CERTAIN RULES AND RESTRICTIONS FOR FIRST-TIME ENROLLEES?

No. But you should take steps to prepare to enroll ahead of time, in the year that you turn 65. First-timers are able to enroll during a seven-month period that begins three months before you turn 65, includes your birthday month, and ends three months after you turn 65. So if your birthday is between May and December, you should plan to enroll during the fall/winter period of that same year.

Depending on your particular situation, you may have some flexibility in choosing a Medicare plan for the first time. There are also special circumstances that may allow you to join or switch plans outside of the formal enrollment period (if you move, for instance, are diagnosed with a chronic condition, or lose employer-based coverage). If you're uncertain, contact Medicare or a local senior assistance agency (see No. 12) for help and information.

FIRST-TIME POINTERS

Most people enrolling for the first time should pick a Medicare Part A and Part B plan, which is required before you can buy a Medicare Advantage plan. You can learn more by visiting the Medicare website: Medicare .gov/people-like-me/new-to-medicare/getting-started-with-medicare.html.

NO. 9: WHAT IF YOU DON'T LIKE YOUR PLAN?

There is a "disenrollment" grace period through the middle of February in the year a policy takes effect, during which you can cancel a plan you don't like, go back to traditional Medicare, or even add a Part D drug-plan. But that grace period only applies to certain drug plans.

NO. 10: WHAT IS THE "DONUT HOLE" IN PRESCRIPTION DRUG COVERAGE, AND IS IT REALLY CLOSING UNDER OBAMACARE?

Yes and no. ObamaCare requires health and drug plans to provide new discounts on generic and brand-name drugs for seniors to close the infamous "donut hole" coverage gap, which kicks in when consumers reach a certain level. Between now and 2020, those discounts and insurance coverage levels will continue to rise, as costs borne by seniors who fall into the gap will shrink.

But the picture of overall drug costs is complicated. For instance, Medicare prescription drug costs were flat or down slightly in 2014 plans, compared to the year before, according to data released by the federal government. The government said the average per-beneficiary Medicare drug costs fell four percent in 2013 and by an additional four percent in 2014.

The federal Centers for Medicare and Medicaid Services (CMS), which administers Medicare, estimated the standard annual plan deductible to be $310 in 2014, down from $325 in 2013. Part D premiums have also been flat for several years, ranging from $37 to $40. The moderation in drug costs is partly tied to slowdown in health-care expenditures, as well as a shift to less-expensive generic drugs.

In 2013, seniors falling into the "donut hole," when spending on drugs, including what individuals and insurers pay, reached that threshold at about $2,970. At that point, seniors were responsible for 50 percent of brand-name drug costs (less than in prior years, as a result of the Affordable Care Act), until drug costs exceeded $4,750, at which time coverage resumed.

For 2014 plans, the rules were changed so the donut hole threshold on combined spending was set at $2,850 ($120 less than in 2013) and the out-of-pocket maximum was lowered to $4,550 (down $200 from the year before).

But that's not all. The share of costs borne by seniors who fall into the gap is also shrinking. Before 2010, seniors in the gap paid all drug costs. Now under ObamaCare, they pay half of those costs out-of-pocket for brand-name drugs (79 percent for cheaper generics), with insurers and discounts from pharmaceutical manufacturers picking up the balance.

The bottom line: Seniors are paying less and the donut hole is shrinking, but Medicare beneficiaries will still have to shoulder a declining percentage of out-of-pocket costs to cover the gap in drug coverage until 2020, when the seniors' donut-hole costs will fall to 25 percent.

NO. 11: WHAT IS SUPPLEMENTAL MEDICARE COVERAGE AND DO YOU NEED IT?

In September 2012, Mt. Sinai researchers released a startling analysis of Medicare coverage that found one in four seniors over the age of 65 exhaust their life savings on out-of-pocket healthcare costs not covered by the federal healthcare program in the last five years of their lives. That means a huge portion of healthcare dollars are spent at the end of seniors' lives and, for many, the cost of dying in the United States far exceeds a lifetime of savings.

The study, published in the *Journal of General Internal Medicine*, found those with dementia or Alzheimer's disease spent the most, averaging $66,155 — twice as much as cancer or GI patients — and that the average costs were well over $38,000.

"I think a lot of people will be surprised by how high these out-of-pocket costs are in the last years of life," said Amy Kelley, an assistant professor of geriatrics and palliative medicine at Mount Sinai School of Medicine in New York City, who led the study.

She noted the findings underscore the fact that, for many, Medicare falls short of one of its key goals: to reduce risk of personal financial catastrophe due to out-of-pocket healthcare expenses. Kelley's analysis, which was based on information from the national Health and Retirement Study, found that one-quarter of seniors spend more than their baseline total household assets, and 43 percent spent more than their non-housing assets.

"The Medicare program provides a significant amount of healthcare coverage to people over 65, but it does not cover co-pays, deductibles, homecare services, or most nursing home care — and these expenses can add up, leading to considerable financial risk from out-of-pocket healthcare expenses," Kelley noted. "Disease-related differences in this risk complicate efforts to anticipate or plan for health-related costs."

Several months later, Kelley published a follow-up study that found Medicare patients enrolled in hospice receive better care at significantly lower costs than those who don't. The study calculated a savings to Medicare of $6.4 million for every 1,000 Medicare beneficiaries who enroll in hospice in the weeks prior to death.

So what does that mean for you? First, you should consider getting supplemental Medicare insurance (a Medigap plan) to cover those uncovered costs right now. Secondly, it's going to be important to look ahead, because Medicare cutbacks under ObamaCare will trim $716 billion from the program over the next decade, which may increase out-of-pocket costs for many beneficiaries.

"The estimate for non-covered items under Medicare could easily exceed $250,000 for a couple," notes Harriet J. Brackey, CFP®, co-chief investment officer with GSK Wealth Advisors, a wealth-management firm in Hollywood, Florida, with $170 million under management.

"I think [supplemental insurance] is absolutely necessary," adds Brackey. "You want to look at it not just in terms of what your premium is, but also what it covers, because some of them look cheap-cheap-cheap and some look expensive. But if you look at what your needs are, you will make a better choice."

Steve Lewit, Investment Advisor Representative, Registered Financial Consultant, and CEO of Wealth Financial Group in Chicago, agrees, noting Medicare recipients can work with health insurance agents, including some who specialize in Medicare services and can also help seniors pick an appropriate supplemental Medicare plan, taking into account individual needs and regional differences in healthcare costs. Senior advocacy groups, such as AARP (formerly referred to as the American Association of Retired People), offer assistance as well: AARP.org, (888) OUR-AARP, (877) 434-7598, (TTY).

Medigap supplement plans will typically cover at least some of your co-pays, deductibles, and other out-of-pocket fees that arise in Medicare. They carry premiums that range from $100 to $1,000 per month, depending on what's covered, your age, and health status. To evaluate your Medigap options, visit Medicare.gov and click on "Health Plans & Medigap Policies" or call (800) 633-4227.

If you sign up for a Medigap policy during your initial Medicare enrollment period, it remains in effect as long as you keep it current, making them essential for people who have pre-existing conditions or require a lot of medical care. Some policies also cover care outside the US, making them especially attractive to people who travel a lot.

In addition to considering a Medigap policy to cover out-of-pocket healthcare costs, Lewit advises Medicare recipients to explore strategies for managing other investment and spending plans for a more "holistic" approach to personal financial planning.

"If I'm going to have to pay more for my healthcare, I've got to bring my taxes down, I have to bring costs for my portfolio down," he says. "You have to watch your costs on other parts of your budget.

"My message for people is now, more than ever, you have to manage your finances holistically — you can't do it piecemeal.

You may be able to save in other areas of your life to compensate for healthcare spending. The ultimate goal of financial planning is to maintain your quality of life, or increase it, so if you have to spend more on healthcare you have to spend less somewhere else or find the right way to reduce costs for all aspects of your financial plan."

NO. 12: WHERE CAN YOU GET UNBIASED HELP AND INFORMATION?

For more information about your options, Medicare administrators have developed a 138-page booklet, "Medicare & You: 2014," which is available at Medicare.gov/Pubs/pdf/10050.pdf. Once you order the handbook, you'll get a copy in the mail every year from Medicare, and may also be contacted by various drug plans.

To sign up for Medicare:

Online: Go to Medicare.gov and click on "Apply online for Medicare now," then follow the instructions on how to prepare your information, apply, complete, and follow up on your application.

In person: Sign up for parts A and B at any Social Security office. To find your local Social Security office, call (800) 772-1213 or enter your zip code at SSA.gov/locator.

By phone: Call (800) 772-1213, or (800) 325-0778 (TTY).

FOR HELP EVALUATING YOUR OPTIONS UNDER MEDICARE:

Medicare: For a consumer's guide to Medicare assembled by federal officials who run the program, go to Medicare.gov and click on "Medicare Basics."

Medicare Plan Comparison Tool: Go to Medicare.gov and click on "Find Health & Drug Plans," or call a Medicare counselor at (800) 633-4227 to help you fill out a worksheet and choose a plan.

Insurers: You can also seek information about a particular health plan through a provider or insurer, but be aware the companies may have a biased view.

FOR INDEPENDENT INFORMATION ON MEDICARE:

State Health Insurance Assistance Program: A range of non-profit and nonbiased agencies and organizations are available to help seniors in all 50 states and the District of Columbia through the State Health Insurance Assistance Program (SHIP) — a national program that offers one-on-one counseling and assistance to people with Medicare and their families. Appendix A lists state-by-state, SHIP program contact information.

Kaiser Family Foundation: For a comprehensive primer on the key elements of Medicare: KFF.org/medicare/issue-brief/medicare-a-primer/.

Medicare Rights Center: For answers to common questions about your rights as a Medicare recipient: MedicareInteractive.org, or call (800) 333-4114.

Center for Medicare Advocacy: For resources to help you resolve a Medicare-related dispute: MedicareAdvocacy.org, or call (860) 456-7790.

AARP: For assistance in picking a plan, a donut-hole calculator, and other aspects of Medicare: AARP.org, or call (888) OUR-AARP, or (888) 687-2277.

Allsup: For help evaluating Medicare options, you can speak with an agent at Allsup, a nationwide provider of Social Security disability and Medicare services, by calling (866) 521-7655 or visiting Medicare.Allsup.com.

NO. 13: WILL CUTS TO MEDICARE ADVANTAGE DOOM THE PROGRAM?
When the Obama Administration proposed reductions in government payments for Medicare Advantage insurance plans — pegged at $11 billion by an insurance industry trade group — many insurers suggested it was more evidence the program might face a tough future.

"These changes will disrupt coverage for Medicare Advantage beneficiaries at a time when evidence clearly demonstrates that Medicare Advantage provides higher-quality care than the fee-for-service part of Medicare," said Karen Ignagni, president of America's Health Insurance Plans, in a statement.

What was left unsaid: The trims announced by the Centers for Medicare and Medicaid Services were only the latest sign that the nation's 14 million Medicare Advantage recipients — nearly one in four Medicare recipients — will shoulder an increasing share of healthcare costs as more Americans become eligible for the program and funding levels shrink.

The new proposal not only included cuts in payment rates for Medicare Advantage, but also trims in levels of profits that insurers can earn, known as Medical Loss Ratios, on Medicare Advantage and Medicare prescription plans.

Under Medicare Advantage, CMS pays insurers a set fee per recipient, which is then passed on to doctors who provide services (unlike traditional Medicare reimbursements paid directly to doctors, based on services they provide).

The changes in Medicare Advantage are part of ObamaCare and represented an eight percent reduction in total for 2014 payments from 2013. In response, many of the nation's major insurers suggested they may pull out of the Medicare Advantage market.

Prior to the 2014 cuts, the Congressional Budget Office estimated seniors with Medicare Advantage plans were already getting about $68 less a month in benefits because of ObamaCare.

Ironically, perhaps, the Medicare Advantage program was designed to open up Medicare to private insurers to control costs, boost completion, and make better use of tax dollars, while providing seniors with additional benefits beyond standard Medicare coverage.

Senior citizens usually need more than traditional Medicare, which typically covers about 60 percent of their medical expenses. Those who can afford to buy Medigap coverage as a supplement, but for those with lower incomes, Medicare Advantage has offered another option to help with copays, coinsurance, and even cover hearing aids or gym memberships.

Over the next decade, ObamaCare proposes to trim $136 billion dollars out of the Medicare Advantage budget.

While the long-term impacts are hard to predict, some insurers are likely to pull out of the market, while others may simply cut benefits and/or raise premiums — trends that have already started to occur.

NO. 14: IS A STAND-ALONE MEDICARE PART D DRUG PLAN RIGHT FOR YOU?

Nearly one in four seniors have chosen to go with a stand-alone Medicare Part D drug plan, which can be purchased along with traditional Medicare or Private Fee-for-Service plans. Premiums typically range in cost from about $15 to $130 per month and deductibles can top $300, according to PlanPrescriber.com, an online insurance agency.

Medicare beneficiaries can choose among two options for prescription drug coverage:

- **Medicare Part D Prescription Drug Plans** are stand-alone policies offered by private insurers and approved by Medicare. They can be added to traditional Medicare coverage, Medicare Supplement (or Medigap) plans, or even Medicare Advantage plans. Anyone enrolled in Medicare Part A or Medicare Part B is eligible for a Part D plan.

- **Medicare Advantage Prescription Drug Plans** are health plans that offer prescription drug coverage to beneficiaries enrolled in both Medicare Part A and Part B.

The huge number and wide variety of Medicare Part D stand-alone drug plans make it difficult for many seniors to determine which plan offers the best coverage. You must compare dozens, or even hundreds of plans in some states, and take into consideration the drugs you take, out-of-pocket costs, pharmacy availability, limitations on certain drugs, and other factors.

When Medicare Part D plans entered the market in 2006, advocates trumpeted the new choices they afforded seniors in picking a drug plan. But what they didn't emphasize was just how MANY choices seniors would have, and how complicated it would make picking a plan.

In most states, the 13 million seniors with Part D plans have dozens of options to choose from. In states with large senior populations, such as Florida and California, Medicare recipients have to pore over more than 100 plans to identify the best deals.

An eye-opening 2013 study revealed just how complicated those choices can be — with even doctors in training having trouble sifting through insurance options to pick the cheapest available plan.

For the study, researchers at the Virginia Commonwealth University School of Medicine in Richmond asked 70 medical students and residents to pick the cheapest plan for a hypothetical patient, "Bill," from a list plans. For each option, the students were given information about monthly premiums, deductibles, network pharmacies, and the estimated annual cost.

The results, published in the Public Library of Science journal, *PLOS ONE*, found that fewer than half of the students correctly chose the plan with the lowest cost. What's more, the researchers found that the more choices students were given, the harder it was to make a good decision about which plan to pick. On average, participants chose a higher cost plans that would have "Bill" spending about $100 more than necessary each year.

The findings are particularly troubling for older people on fixed incomes who may have more difficulty understanding the costs than younger med students and residents. Seniors tend to place an emphasis on total cost in picking a plan, but some policies cover certain drugs differently, and those levels change year to year. Throughout the nation, 1,169 Part D plans were available in 2014, according to the Kaiser Family Foundation.

The researchers called on Medicare administrators to selectively contract with fewer plans, reduce the number of options, or present less information about each plan. CMS officials could also estimate which drug plan would be cheapest for beneficiaries and automatically enroll them. But unless, or until, such changes are made, seniors have no choice but to become savvy consumers or work with insurance specialists or patient advocates.

Allsup, a nationwide Social Security Disability Insurance (SSDI) representation company and Medicare advisory organization, notes that many seniors don't use the open enrollment period to compare and contrast their choices, primarily because of the complexities of the plans.

Only 15 percent of seniors report changing their Medicare plans each year, even though doing so could save them money, according to a 2013 Allsup survey of seniors, using data collected in 2012. In fact, 43 percent of seniors said they have experienced unexpected costs for medications, treatments, and doctor visits that Medicare did not pick up, according to the Allsup survey.

"Comparing plans and choosing coverage can be complex," said Paula Muschler, operations manager of the Allsup Medicare Advisor plan, an Allsup service offering personalized help that includes customized research and enrollment assistance. "As a result many people stay where they are, missing out on important benefits and cost savings, rather than deal with the complexity.

"Medicare plans can change what they cover, or your own needs may have changed, or both. If you continue with the same plan next year, you could find your plan doesn't cover things you thought it did or that you need, leaving you holding the bill."

Here are a few reasons why beneficiaries should review their Medicare plans during the annual, open-enrollment season and consider switching plans:

- **Change in health.** If you have developed a health condition in the previous 12 months that requires a new drug or specialist's care you should determine if another plan would better cover your needs.

- **A move or planned move.** With the exception of traditional Medicare, most Medicare plans have geographic restrictions. If you plan to move, be sure to check plans in the new area of residence for one that best suits your needs.

- **Change in healthcare providers.** With changes in Medicare funding and ObamaCare, many doctors, hospitals, and healthcare providers may change their policies on Medicare patients. Some physicians may retire or relocate, and medical facilities may change their terms. Be sure your plan continues to cover visits to your doctor and facilities in your health-provider network.

- **Change in plan coverage.** Plans can alter the drugs, procedures, and conditions they cover. Premiums, co-pays, or deductibles are increasing for many plans and occur year to year. Be sure any plan you have continues to meet your needs and what you will pay in the coming year. Alternative plans may offer more complete coverage with lower costs available in your area.

- **Also worth noting:** If you already have some form of pre-scription-drug coverage from an employer- or union-sponsored plan, Medigap coverage, or a program for veterans for federal workers, you might not need to join a Medicare prescription-drug plan and, in fact, your coverage may be better than what you would receive through a Part D policy.

NO. 15: MEDICARE SCAMS AND HOW TO AVOID THEM

ObamaCare doesn't directly affect Medicare in terms of enrollment, sign up and administration of the program. But security experts and identity theft specialists are warning that many scams have emerged across the country as con artists attempt to take advantage of the confusion that many seniors may have about the Affordable Care Act and its impact on Medicare.

"Confusion about what exactly the Affordable Care Act means for consumers and businesses is what con artists prey upon," said Karen Nalven, president of the Better Business Bureau serving West Florida. "Scammers' favorite tools are confusion and fear."

Federal Trade Commission Chairwoman Edith Ramirez claimed that federal officials are cracking down on ObamaCare-related scams, particularly those aimed at seniors and Medicare recipients, but fraud abuse remains rampant. Former Health and Human Services secretary Kathleen Sebelius also noted regulators have added safeguards to protect consumers from health-insurance fraud.

"We are sending a clear message that we will not tolerate anyone seeking to defraud consumers in the Health Insurance Marketplace," Sebelius said. "We have strong security safeguards in the marketplace to protect people's personal information against fraud and we will work with our partners to aggressively prosecute bad actors, just as we have been doing in Medicare, Medicaid, and the Children's Health Insurance Program."

Here are some common Medicare scams and how to protect yourself:

- **Bogus ObamaCare cards**. The Better Business Bureau reports numerous complaints from seniors who have received phone calls from individuals claiming to be government officials offering new health insurance cards they say are required by ObamaCare. Consumers are asked to provide bank account and social security numbers to claim their card. But the truth is, there's no such thing as an ObamaCare card.

Scammers have also been requesting personal information in exchange for a government-issued, ObamaCare card. "This is the latest twist on the 'Medicare scam' that BBB has seen for years," said the BBB's Nalven. "Whenever there is a new government program or new public policy, fraudsters will take advantage of people. But the simple fact is there is no Affordable Care card. It's a scam."

- **Fake government employee solicitations.** Authorities in Florida, California, and other states with large senior populations have reported cases of con artists offering to help sign up older residents on Medicare for coverage through ObamaCare.

Callers say they need to confirm the identity of the folks they call and ask for Social Security numbers and medical info. The scammers bank on many seniors falsely believing Medicare benefits are changing under ObamaCare (they aren't). Some seniors are also confused by overlapping sign-up periods for Medicare in the last two months of the year.

- **Medicare scare ploys.** AARP has received many complaints from people over 65 who were phoned by individuals claiming they are about to lose their Medicare coverage or that ObamaCare is replacing their plans — and asking for their Social Security number and other private information to keep their plans intact. But such claims are not true. In fact, it's unlawful for insurers to sell an ObamaCare health exchange policy to anyone on Medicare.

TO PROTECT YOURSELF:

- Medicare beneficiaries need to know they don't have to do anything differently as a result of ObamaCare, and will continue to go to Medicare.gov to sign up for plans.

- The new ObamaCare Health Insurance Exchanges are only for people who don't qualify for Medicare, Medicaid, or get insurance through their employer. Those individuals can sign up for health insurance through the exchanges by visiting HealthCare.gov, or calling (800) 318-2596.

- Federal agencies rarely contact Medicare recipients by phone — they typically use mail instead. So if you receive a phone solicitation, hang up immediately.

- Never give out personal information, and if you have mistakenly provided information to someone you think is trying to rip you off, contact your bank, credit card providers and the three major credit bureaus — TransUnion, Experian, and Equifax — to monitor for potential identity thieves.

In summary, as you near eligibility, are new to the system, or are already fully indoctrinated, take the time to review the following Medicare considerations:

DaVINCI DO'S

- If you're a Medicare recipient or approaching the age of eligibility, be sure to take the time to come up with a game plan for picking a policy that suits your needs. You need to evaluate not only costs and prices, but also whether your doctors are part of the plan, what prescription medicines are paid for (and not), and what extra benefits — eye exams, dental care, wellness visits, and even "Silver Sneakers" health club memberships — are covered.

- Get help. Check the federal website — Medicare.gov — for general information and enrollment. But it's also a good idea to consult one of the many consumer-advocacy organizations that provide assistance to seniors looking for help in choosing a Medicare plan, such as AARP (AARP .org/health, 888-687-2277). Another good place to start is your State Health Insurance Assistance Program (state-by-state contact information is available in Appendix A, or visit SHIPTalk.org).

- Find out if you qualify for a discount. If you are on a limited income and have few assets, you could qualify for help with all or part of your Medicare premiums, deductibles, co-payments, or prescription drug costs. Individuals with incomes under $17,505 and assets less than $13,440, and couples with incomes under $23,595 and assets less than $26,860 qualify for subsidies. People who have chronic health conditions — such as heart disease, cancer, and diabetes, or live in nursing homes may also qualify for special needs assistance. For more information, contact Social Security at (800) 772-1213 or go to SocialSecurity.gov.

DaVINCI DON'TS

- If you currently have a Medicare plan, don't make the common mistake of simply renewing your policy year-to-year without checking to be sure your plan hasn't changed. Before being locked in, check what's called a "Notice of Change," supplied by your insurer, for any alterations in costs, premiums, coverage levels, doctor and hospital networks, and other benefits for the next year. It's also a good idea to at least shop around and see what's offered by other plans, for comparison. You may be able to get a better deal by making a switch.

- Don't overlook the possibility that you will need to buy a private "Medigap" supplement policy or a Medicare Advantage plan to cover out-of-pocket expenses not covered by their policies, including deductibles, co-payments, and other costs. To evaluate your Medigap options, visit Medicare.gov and click on "Health Plans & Medigap Policies," or call (800) 633-4227.

- Never give your Medicare information or other personal info, such as your Social Security number, to anyone you don't know who claims to need it in order to continue your coverage (particularly over the phone) under the new mandates of the Affordable Care Act. Many scams have emerged across the country as con artists attempt to take advantage of confusion many seniors may have about the Affordable Care Act and its impact on Medicare.

Thinking Through the Unthinkable

IT'S THE NIGHTMARE scenario no one sees coming: An accident or illness leaves you unable to make decisions on your own — about your health, your healthcare, your finances, your assets, and other aspects of your life.

The truth is no one wants to think about a life-threatening condition or their own death, let alone plan for it. That's why the vast majority of Americans don't have advance directives, including a living will, that spell out their end-of-life wishes should they become incapacitated and unable to speak for themselves.

Just 26.3 percent of US residents have completed advance directives, according to a 2013 study published in the *American Journal of Preventive Medicine* based on national surveys involving nearly 8,000 Americans. It found advance directives are more likely to be completed by women, whites, married people, individuals with chronic conditions, and those with a college education. But the results also showed the three out of four Americans who have not taken steps to document their end-of-life wishes don't know what is legally required to do so.

The findings echoed a 2011 Associated Press-Life Goes Strong poll found that 64 percent of baby boomers don't have a living will or other advance directives, and have not named a person to speak on their behalf should they become unable to do so. (Surveys. AP.org/data%5CKnowledgeNetworks%5CAP_Boomers%20Only_ Topline_062111.pdf.)

Without such advance directives, questions about how doctors, hospitals, and other facilities handle your care — if you are unable to communicate — could set the stage for a painful legal and medical battle over your fate that could you leave and your family members in a lurch.

Case in point: Terri Schiavo, a Florida woman whose end-of-life care sparked a protracted family feud that ultimately made its way to the US Supreme Court and the halls of Congress. In 1990, at age 26, Schiavo's heart stopped beating, leaving her with irreversible brain damage and in a permanent vegetative state. With no end-of-life care instructions from Schiavo in writing, her husband sought legal authority to allow her to die with dignity, arguing that was what Schiavo would have wanted. But her parents filed suit to keep her alive. Eventually, the courts allowed Schiavo's feeding tube to be removed in 2005 and she died two weeks later.

Individuals on both sides of the debate over Schiavo's care agreed on few issues, but nearly all involved say her case makes a strong argument for drafting a living will and other healthcare directives.

Such documents aren't just for older adults. An unexpected health emergency can strike at any age (as Schiavo's case attests). Regardless of whether you are healthy and young, or older and living with a chronic or life-threatening condition, placing your wishes in writing can help ensure that you will receive the medical treatment you would like to have if you end up in such a situation. Doing so can also save your loved ones a world of pain, difficulty, and expense.

The good news is that advance directives can be simple — merely declaring you don't want "heroic measures" be taken to prolong your life — or they can be more involved and identify specific procedures you would like to be taken, or not (such as resuscitation, but not life-support, feeding or breathing tubes).

But the key is to be sure they are legal and can hold up against any challenges or complications that may emerge in a crisis. To help you get started, here are 10 questions and answers about living wills and other advance directives.

No. 1: What Is a Living Will?

In simplest terms, a living will is a written document that details your wishes for medical care if you end up in what is legally known as a "persistent vegetative state" — from which there is virtually no chance of recovery — after an injury or illness, and you are unable to communicate. Each state has its own regulations and forms for living wills.

"I typically tell prospective clients that the living will applies to one situation: You are in a persistent vegetative state as defined by Florida statutes and you cannot be maintained without extraordinary means (breathing tube, feeding tube, etc.)," says David Netburn, an attorney who specializes in estate planning and healthcare-related legal matters in Coral Springs, Florida. "The living will says that if I am in such a state, I do not wish to be maintained and I am empowering the person named therein to speak for me and tell the medical professionals my wishes."

"The common misconception here is that you are giving someone discretion to 'pull the plug.' This is not the case. You have already decided for yourself that you do not wish to be maintained and all the person you name in the document is empowered to do is tell the doctors your decision."

A living will provides a guide for the types of medical treatments and life-sustaining measures you want — and don't want. It can include specific provisions on mechanical breathing devices (respiration and ventilation), feeding tubes, and do-not-resuscitate orders that essentially guarantee that no extraordinary measures are taken to keep you alive via life-support.

While a living will doesn't always require an attorney's involvement, the cost to have a lawyer draft one — to guarantee its validity — is typically minimal. It's a good idea to give copies to at least a few close relatives, friends, or colleagues, so your wishes are well-known. You might even discuss your desires with your doctor or healthcare professionals involved in your care.

No. 2: What Is a Healthcare Proxy?

Living wills provide a guide to the wishes for your end-of-life care, but they are intended to apply in only a very specific scenario — in the event you fall into a persistent vegetative state. That's why it is even more important to complete and sign a "healthcare designation" that identifies an individual as your healthcare proxy to make medical decisions for you, if necessary, so there is no confusion or question over who should make any difficult judgment calls about your care if you can't do so on your own.

Such individuals are given what are sometimes referred to as durable healthcare powers of attorney (POA) that grant them the authority to speak on your behalf.

Netburn adds that in, many ways, designating a healthcare proxy is more important than crafting a living will.

"The healthcare designation, which is also referred to as a healthcare proxy in other states, is a document which enables the person named therein to give informed consent for the person signing the document. It is critical because the situations in which it could be utilized are far more likely to come up than the Living Will [can anticipate]," notes Netburn.

"For example, [if] you are involved in a car accident and taken by ambulance to the ER, I expect that most ERs will administer emergency medical treatment. But what happens if you are admitted, unconscious, and in need of further medical treatment? Here, there is a need for someone to be able to give informed consent in order for you to have such treatment. This is where the healthcare designation is critical. It allows the person you have named to give informed consent when you are unable to do so for yourself. In the absence of having a valid healthcare designation, the patient's family may have to hire a lawyer and file an Emergency Guardianship Proceeding which is time-consuming, expensive and avoidable."

In designating a medical POA, you should make sure to consult the person ahead of time, and it's a good idea to share your decision with other close relatives or friends who might presume they have some say about your care (particularly if they are likely to

HEALTHCARE POA

Healthcare powers of attorney only concern your medical treatment and are independent of POA designations authorizing someone to make financial or legal decisions on your behalf.

have religious views or other perspectives that might put them in conflict with your own end-of-life wishes).

Netburn also recommends creating a "HIPAA Release," clearing the way for your healthcare-designate to communicate with your healthcare providers about your care. HIPAA — short for the Health Insurance Portability and Accountability Act of 1996 — is a medical privacy statute that bars doctors from discussing details of your medical history and care with others without your permission.

"It is my practice to do a HIPAA Release for each client we prepare healthcare-related documents for so that the medical professionals who treat the patient can speak freely with the persons named in the healthcare related documents," he says. "It would be pointless to be the person named in the healthcare designation or living will but have medical professionals refuse to talk to you because of HIPAA concerns."

"Everyone over 18 should have the healthcare designation and HIPAA Release done. Most people will also do a living will. Sometimes people will have a philosophical opposition to the living will, but my experience has been that most people do one."

No. 3: Can Your Medical POA Be a Non-Relative?

Yes. You can choose any person to act as your healthcare proxy. For instance, you might feel that it may be too emotionally taxing for a spouse, partner, adult children, siblings, or parents to carry out your wishes. You may also want the person in charge or your healthcare to be different from the agent you choose to handle your financial or legal affairs.

Here are some factors to consider, when choosing a medical POA:

- The person you choose should understand your wishes, and have the ability to make decisions that honor them above all, even if challenged by family members, friends, or healthcare professionals.

- It's a good idea to choose someone who lives near your residence or at least in your home state. "Proximity may matter when informed consent is needed now," Netburn notes.

- Your medical POA should able to make difficult decisions dispassionately, without succumbing to emotional or irrational choices, in difficult situations. Sound out a potential proxy by asking how comfortable he or she would be to take on such a responsibility. Do not to pick someone merely out of feelings of guilt or a sense of obligation.

- Be sure your healthcare proxy does not subscribe to any religious, cultural, or personal beliefs that would prevent them from carrying out your wishes.

- When contemplating a healthcare proxy, it might help ask yourself the following questions: Who among your family and friends is able to handle high-pressure situations with confidence and intelligence? With whom have you regularly had candid conversations about difficult topics? Who is most likely to make a tough call that is truly in your best interest, regardless of the consequences (such as opposition from other family members)?

- Consider selecting an alternate proxy, just in case your primary POA is unavailable or is otherwise incapable of carrying out the directives in your living will. For instance, designating your spouse or partner as your POA could complicate matters if you are both left incapacitated by a car accident and there is no designated alternate proxy to help guide decisions. "Always have two layers, if possible," Netburn recommends.

No. 4: What Treatments Would You Want — and Not Want?

It may be the toughest question you'll ever have to answer: Under what circumstances would you want to allow for nature to simply take its course without medical intervention to save your life? We all die, of course. But end-of-life decisions are often complicated and difficult. Without knowing what specific situations you may encounter, it can be difficult to say what you would and would not want done in terms of care, treatments, and procedures, in a way that can cover every end-of-life situation.

But it's important to consider your personal values in determining your wishes. For instance, would you want to stay alive at all costs, regardless of your ability to make decisions on your own and the potentially staggering costs of institutional long-term care? At what point would you say life would not be worth living? If there is no possibility of a cure, or halting or reversing the progress of a terminal condition, would you want to extend your treatment? When would you want your healthcare providers to shift from life-saving treatments to palliative care, which does not aim to prolong your life, but aims to ease any pain or discomfort associated with a terminal illness or injury?

In poring over your options, it can help to talk with your doctor, a counselor, faith-based individual, or anyone else you think would be helpful about the following matters:

- **Do-not-resuscitate (DNR) order.** This document registers your desire not to have medical personnel perform extraordinary measures, such as cardiopulmonary resuscitation (CPR), if your heart stops or if you stop breathing. You don't have to include a DNR order in any advance-directive documents you create, and you don't need a living will to have a DNR order. You can simply have your doctor put a DNR order in your medical records to make your desires clear.

- **Resuscitation.** Under what circumstances would you want to be resuscitated — and not — by cardiopulmonary resuscitation (CPR), or by a defibrillation device that shocks the heart after it has stopped beating?

- **Mechanical ventilation.** When, and for how long, would you want an artificial, mechanical respirator to take over your breathing if you're unable to do so on your own?

- **Nutritional assistance.** If you become unable to eat or drink, and the only way you could survive would be through an intravenous or stomach tube that supplies your body with nutrients and fluids, for how long, if at all, would you want to be nourished in this way?

- **Dialysis.** Kidney failure is often the first step toward death in terminal patients. Dialysis can take over for the function of your kidneys, removing waste from your blood and managing fluid levels after they stop working. When — and for how long — you would want to receive this treatment. The same is true for other procedures, such as blood transfusions.

- **Brain death.** For many terminal patients, such as those in what are called persistent vegetative states, brain function falls to minimal or immeasurable levels and they never regain consciousness. Yet for some, the physical body can continue to function with artificial life-support systems for years, with virtually no hope of recovery. Under what circumstances, would you choose to simply be allowed to die if your brain function were deemed minimal or indeterminable?

- **Organ donation.** Advance directives can spell out any wishes you have about donating your organs and tissues for transplantation — something you should consider doing, regardless of your wishes, in light of the tens of thousands of Americans who die every year waiting for an organ for transplant surgery. You can also donate your body for scientific study; contact a nearby medical school or your doctor for details.

No. 5: Why Do You Need To Put It in Writing?

Every state has its own laws on advance directives, so it's important for you to find out what's required in your home state and put your wishes in writing, using appropriate forms and statements. State-based forms are available from a variety of organizations, such as the National Hospice and Palliative Care Organization (NHPCO.org, 703-837-1500), and you may want to consult an attorney if you're confused about what you need to do to comply with your state's requirements.

"In Florida the documents must be signed in the presence of two witnesses and it is our practice to have the signature acknowledged before a notary public," Netburn points out. "I have seen that some lawyers in other states combine the living will and healthcare designation in one document with different provisions for the different situations. I would suggest a lawyer who practices in the area of estate planning in the state where you reside to ensure that the documents are compliant with state law both as to form and execution."

After filling out the forms, make sure to give copies to your doctor, healthcare proxy, relatives, and (if appropriate) close friends. You should also keep a copy with your other important personal papers. Some people even keep a card in their purse or wallet indicating they have a living will, a contact name and phone number, and/or their doctor's contact information.

While such documents are typically considered an important part of end-of-life planning, Netburn argues they should be drafted for everyone over the age of 18.

"The notion that these healthcare-related documents are only necessary for the elderly that is a fallacy," he says. "Tragedy can strike at any age and why add insult to injury and have to file an Emergency Guardianship Proceeding in order for a loved one to get the care he/she needs?

"An interesting sidebar here is [that I recently] did healthcare-related documents for a husband and wife and then separate healthcare-related documents for their 18-year-old daughter who was going off to college. As the daughter had reached the age of majority, her parents could no longer give informed consent as her legal guardians."

No. 6: Should You Update Your Advance Directives Periodically?

Yes. A number of circumstances should prompt you to review and, if necessary, update your advance directives. The rule of thumb: Living wills should be updated whenever you would update a last will and testament. Some examples:

- Changes in state and federal laws on living wills, power-of-attorney provisions, and other regulations on end-of-life care.

- Any change in the status of your health, such as a diagnosis of a life-threatening condition, or if you are facing the possibility of an upcoming surgery or hospitalization.

- A change of heart about how you want any end-of-life decisions handled.

- Moving to a new state, where regulations and laws may be different.

- Major changes in life or family status, such as a divorce or new marriage, or an alteration in your relationship with your healthcare proxy.

Updating your advance directives is as simple as getting new forms to fill out and discussing the changes with your doctor, family, and friends (and providing updated copies to those to whom you have given earlier versions).

No. 7: Can Your Healthcare-Related Documents Be Invalidated or Challenged as Faulty?

Yes. Under certain conditions, the terms of your advance directives can be challenged legally. For instance, in most states you must be over the age of 18, and be considered a legal adult, to have a living will.

Advance directives can also be invalidated if it can be determined that you were mentally incapacitated or not of "sound mind" when you crafted them. In addition, they can be challenged if you were coerced into making them or in designating your healthcare proxy.

The key point here is that no one should be allowed to make decisions for you on such matters.

No. 8: Can Your Doctor Refuse Any of Your Advance Directives?

Yes. It is rare, but occasionally a doctor may have ethical, moral, or religious reasons that prevent him from following the directives in your living will.

Your best hedge against such a possibility is to have an in-depth discussion with your doctor ahead of time about the details in your living will. It's also a good idea to ask candidly about any reservations he or she might have, for any reason, about acting on your wishes.

If conflicts emerge, it might be time to find a new physician who will place your wishes, desires, and beliefs about end-of-life decisions first.

No. 9: Are There Other Documents You Might Need to Be Sure Your Wishes Are Carried Out After You're Gone?

A full estate plan should include healthcare-related documents, but also testamentary documents such as a will and/or trusts. These documents are a blueprint for how you want your affairs settled after you've died. They typically cover the care of your children, your finances, belongings, and anything else of value you may have.

They spell out who should take custody of any under-aged children you have, how and to whom you'd like your property and assets distributed, an executor (or executors) to carry out the terms and conditions of your will, and the handling of any digital assets you have — such as e-mail accounts, social-networking websites such as Facebook, Linkedin, and Twitter accounts, blogs, online backup services, photo and document sharing websites, business accounts, domain names, virtual property, and computer files.

ASSET DISTRIBUTION

If your assets are larger than the current federal estate tax exemption amount ($5,340,000), you may want to consult an accountant and an attorney to maximize the distribution to your heirs.

No. 10: How Can You Help an Older Parent or Relative Make Similar Plans?

Many boomers are not only planning for their own futures, as well as their children's, but they are also playing a leading role in helping their parents or other elderly relatives craft sound end-of-life plans. If you are a part of that sandwiched generation, here are some suggestions for helping your parents identify their wishes on living wills, POA designates, last wills, and other advance directives.

- **Open up a dialogue.** It's a difficult conversation to get started, but it's worth taking the time to consult your parents about how they want their medical, financial, and legal affairs handled if they are no longer able to make decisions on their own. Ask whether they have created a living will or last will and testament, have considered advance directives, designated a healthcare POA, or have any other wishes they'd like to see carried out.

- **Be tactful, but firm on medical care.** Be sensitive to privacy, but ask for personal information about doctors, medicines, medical history, and any other issues that will help you plan for their healthcare and medication needs. NOTE: Before Medicare can disclose personal health information about an elderly relative to you, the person must let Medicare know in writing by filling out a "Medicare Authorization to Disclose Personal Health Information" form. Find one at Medicare.gov.

- **Help them create a living will, healthcare POA.** If they have not created a living will or determined who should have the legal right to make medical and treatment decisions if they are unable to, encourage them to do so by putting them in writing with your help.

- **After-death wishes.** Ask about any other after-death wishes they may have, including details about how they would like their remains handled (cremation, burial, mausoleum internment, donation).

For more information on how to become authorized to make healthcare decisions on an elderly relative's behalf, we recommend:

DaVINCI DO'S

- Create a Personal Health Record (PHR) for the person you're trying to help. A PHR is usually an electronic file or record of health information and recent services, including the person's medical history, hospital records, dates of recent physical exams, major illnesses, operations, allergies, and medicines. Various companies offer PHRs. If the person has Medicare, you can enter the information from My-Medicare.gov into the PHR so it's easier to view in different ways. Visit Medicare.gov to learn more about PHRs and get details on special PHR projects in certain states; check out the Medicare website for a Personal Health Records brochure, or other Medicare publications. (Medicare.gov/Publications/.)

- Learn more about living wills and advance directives. The American Bar Association website offers a wealth of information about living wills, advance directives and healthcare designations. Visit AmericanBar.org. The ABA also provides links to various State Bar Associations, detailing state-specific information at AmericanBar.org/groups/bar_services/resources/state_local_bar_associations.html.

- Be sure that the person that you choose as your medical POA has the ability to carry out your wishes even if challenged by your loved ones, lives nearby to your home or at least in your state, and is able to make difficult decisions without succumbing to emotion.

DaVINCI DON'TS

- Don't go it alone — seek help. Contact your local office on aging, your state health department, or an attorney to learn more about advance directives. You can also visit ElderCare. gov, or call (800) 677-1116 to help find local resources and services that serve the older adults.

- Don't forget to have a HIPPA Release filled out designating your healthcare proxy. The HIPAA form, along with other medical POA documents, will insure complete cooperation from healthcare providers.

- Do not choose your medical POA out of guilt or obligation. Also, don't forget that if choosing a spouse or partner as your proxy, be sure to choose an alternate in the event that both you and your spouse/partner become incapacitated.

The Lifelong Journey to Health

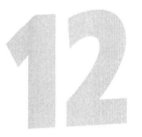

AS A VETERAN CARDIOLOGIST with the renowned Heart MD Institute in Manchester, CT, Dr. Stephen T. Sinatra has seen his share of health trends over the years. But he has also observed a growing tendency among his patients in the past decade or so that he finds troubling: Many are living longer, but aren't exactly what you might call healthy or well.

In fact, for a growing number of his patients, heart disease, diabetes, cancer, high blood pressure, or other chronic conditions are unwelcome companions on the road to old age.

"If you look just at diabetes, there's been an alarming increase over the last few decades," says Dr. Sinatra. "When you have an increase in diabetes you see an increase in heart disease and other conditions. So, yes, we are seeing that trend in our patients."

Dr. Sinatra's practice offers a doc's-eye view of what many experts say is a reality confronting many baby boomers today: Life expectancy has risen to the highest level it's ever been, largely thanks to advances in medical science and dramatic improvements in healthcare in the six decades since the first boomers were born. Yet, at the same time, more Americans are living with chronic ailments — many of them tied to unhealthy lifestyles, bad diets, lack of exercise, smoking, and other disease-causing habits.

Data from the Experts

A recent report card on the nation's wellness by the not-for-profit United Health Foundation underscores what might be called the US Longevity Paradox: *America's Health Rankings* report indicates an American born in 2012 can expect to live 78.5 years — 1.7 years more than in 2000 — but he or she is also more likely to be obese or overweight and suffer from diabetes, cancer, or cardiovascular disease than even a decade ago.

Despite spending more on healthcare per capita than other wealthy nations, the United States trails other affluent countries on a number of health fronts, according to the UHF report:

- More than a quarter of American adults — nearly 28 percent — are clinically obese, which is defined as being at least 30 pounds overweight. That's 66 million people. One reason: About one in four people don't engage in any structured physical activity of any kind.

- The annual medical costs associated with obesity-related diseases alone is a whopping $147 billion.

- The incidence of diabetes has grown to nearly one in 10 Americans — and is rising.

- About 30 percent of the US population has high blood pressure.

- Despite the rise in chronic diseases, the nation's overall death rate has declined markedly since 1990, with premature deaths falling 18 percent overall, cardiovascular deaths down 35 percent, and cancer deaths down 8 percent.

- Health and longevity may vary widely by geography. For instance, Vermont is the healthiest state in the nation, partly due to low rates of infectious diseases and a high rate of health insurance coverage among its residents. Mississippi and Arkansas are the unhealthiest states, largely because of high rates of obesity, diabetes, inactivity, tobacco use, and a low infant birth weight.

The UHF report is based on an examination of 24 measures of health — tobacco and alcohol abuse, exercise, infectious diseases, and cancer and heart disease rates — from the files of the US Centers for Disease Control and Prevention, American Medical Association, Census Bureau, and the Federal Bureau of Investigation.

Reed Tuckson, MD, the medical consultant for United Health Foundation, said the report reflects a significant good-news, bad-news story when it comes to the health of the nation's boomers.

"The good news is we're living longer; the bad news is while we're living longer we're living sicker," he notes. "But it doesn't have to be this way. These are largely preventable illnesses. The point we're making is what's underneath the chronic disease rates, of course, are the risk factors that lead to them. Number one on that list would be tobacco use, closely followed by obesity, with [nearly] 28 percent of the US population obese now and 23 percent of the population exhibiting sedentary lifestyles."

The UHF report's findings aren't the only indications that the baby-boom generation faces a tenuous health future, unless trends change:

- The American Heart Association reported cardiovascular causes still account for one in every three deaths in the US, even though the death rate has fallen by a third since 1999.

- The CDC released a study showing residents of Southern states are most likely to have poor heart health, but that only three percent of all Americans without cardiovascular problems meet the key criteria for heart health — on weight, blood pressure, activity and diet.

- A global health report by Washington University researchers noted great strides have been made in fighting killer diseases, but many nations — including the US — face rising financial costs tied to chronic diseases. The 50-nation study, *Global Burden of Disease*, found malnutrition has dropped as a leading cause of death, but the effects of over-eating are taking its place, with 13 million deaths due to stroke and heart disease — tied to eating and drinking too much, smoking, and inactivity.

- New research by the non-partisan Commonwealth Fund found the United States leads 15 other high-income nations, including Germany, France, and the United Kingdom when it comes to the death rate from such preventable diseases as cancer, diabetes, infections, and heart disease, before age 75. Despite the fact that the United States spends more than double what other nations spend per-person on healthcare, with the American system accounting for nearly one-fifth of the US economy, we still trail the European Union when it comes to preventing deaths. The study, published in the journal *Health Policy*, found the preventable mortality rate in the United States is almost twice that of France — with 96 preventable deaths per 100,000 American residents.

"This study points to substantial opportunity to prevent premature death in the United States. We spend far more than any of the comparison countries — up to twice as much — yet are improving less rapidly," said Commonwealth Fund Senior Vice President Cathy Schoen. "The good news is we know lower death rates are achievable if we enhance access and ensure high-quality care regardless of where you live."

Dr. Tuckson believes the new alarms health experts are sounding should prompt aggressive campaigns — comparable to anti-smoking and polio-eradication initiatives — to change Americans' behaviors as we grow older.

Without a change, the already-stressed US healthcare system won't be able to handle the growing number of seniors — and soon to be seniors — who will need an increased level of care in coming decades, with doctor shortages already emerging in many regions.

One complicating factor: Health experts expect healthcare reforms tied to ObamaCare extending health coverage to up to 46 million additional uninsured Americans — many with largely untreated chronic conditions to this point — will exacerbate the nation's doctor deficits.

According to the Association of American Medical Colleges, the nation now faces a shortage of some 9,000 primary care doctors, including general internists, family doctors, geriatricians, and pediatricians. Over the next 15 years, those shortages will worsen, particularly in rural areas, inner cities, and other areas where fewer doctors practice. That doctor deficit is projected to hit 63,000 by 2015, and will double again by 2025. Shortfalls are also projected for some medical specialists who care for patients with chronic disease.

"The upshot is we are facing a frightening picture in the coming days with an extraordinary burden of diseases pouring into a medical care system that is already over-burdened. So we're talking about two speeding trains heading directly at one another and moving at lightning speed," says Dr. Tuckson.

"I think it is essential that we have affordable healthcare for every American," he adds, citing a key goal of the new healthcare reforms under Obamacare. "But as important as that is, it is more important to prevent disease by addressing these key risk factors. We're putting our emphasis on treatment and medical care; but, we need to work more on prevention of disease. We are all in this together and government cannot do this alone."

Some Hopeful Signs

Not all the news is bad on the national health front, of course. Several promising signs suggest progress is being made toward building a healthier nation.

US rates of smoking and alcohol abuse have declined over the past four decades, with tobacco use falling from 40 percent to 19 percent since 1971, and the share of Americans who drink heavily dropping from seven percent to four percent. And federal statistics show the percentage of people with high blood pressure has plummeted by two-thirds since the 1970s, while those with high cholesterol fell by more than one-third.

"I'm certainly very hopeful that people are starting to get the message. I would never doubt the capacity of the nation to address challenging problems," Dr. Tuckson says. "Cardiovascular death rates and cancer death rates are going down, so we know that medical care can be effective in lengthening our lives. That does help us and we are glad for it, but given the increasing experience with chronic illness, we can't "medicalize" our way out of this problem: prevention is more important than ever!"

His prescription for America is simple: Most people need to move more, eat less, and take more active steps to take better care of themselves.

AMERICA'S HEALTH RANKINGS STATE-BY-STATE

1. Hawaii	14. Washington	27. Kansas	40. Ohio
2. Vermont	15. New York	28. Arizona	41. Indiana
3. Minnesota	16. Maine	29. Pennsylvania	42. Tennessee
4. Massachusetts	17. Wyoming	30. Illinois	43. South Carolina
5. New Hampshire	18. Iowa	31. .Delaware	44. Oklahoma
6. Utah	19. Rhode Island	32. New Mexico	45. Kentucky
7. Connecticut	20. Wisconsin	33. Florida	46. West Virginia
8. Colorado	21. California	34. Michigan	47. Alabama
9. North Dakota	22. South Dakota	35. North Carolina	48. Louisiana
10. New Jersey	23. Montana	36. Texas	49. Arkansas
11. Nebraska	24. Maryland	37. Nevada	50. Mississippi
12. Idaho	25. Alaska	38. Georgia	
13. Oregon	26. Virginia	39. Montana	

Source: United Health Foundation, http://www.americashealthrankings.org/states

"It doesn't need to be more complicated than that," he says. "Just get up and move. Get on a bicycle, walk, garden . . . just do something. Because what we're learning is that if you can just go from no activity at all to just a little bit of activity that will significantly help you, in terms of longevity."

Prescriptions for Health

In light of these dire statistics and predictions on health, what's the best way to stay healthy — mentally and physically — as you grow older? You already know the easier-said-than-done prescription for health: Eat a primarily plant-based diet high in nutrient-rich fruits and vegetables, exercise at least 20 to 30 minutes per day, get a minimum of seven to eight hours of sleep nightly, and manage stress effectively by some means.

But beyond these basics, it's important to know we have control over many aspects of our health — regardless of genetics and environmental factors we can't control — and the choices we make can affect our risks for developing cancer and other serious diseases.

One key to making good choices involves following best-practice recommendations for screening tests that identify cancer, heart disease, diabetes and other chronic conditions so they can be caught and combatted early, when they are more effectively treated, slowed, or even cured.

To help you make healthy choices and understand which screenings you should consider, here is a breakdown of recommendations by age and gender, taken from the latest guidelines from the American Cancer Society, American Heart Association, the Centers for Disease Control and Prevention, and the US Department of Health and Human Services.

Screening Recommendations for Men and Women of All Ages

Old or young. Fat or thin. Man or woman. Healthy or not. There are some things we all can do to boost our health and reduce the risks posed by the nation's "big three" killers: heart disease, cancer, and diabetes. Among them:

AVOID TOBACCO

Studies have repeatedly found there is no safe form or level of tobacco use. If you smoke or chew tobacco, the single biggest step you can take to live a longer, healthier life is to quit. You'll greatly reduce your risk of lung cancer and cardiovascular disease — no matter what age you are or how long you have been using tobacco — and the benefits begin to accrue almost immediately. Need help kicking the habit? Start by calling the American Cancer Society at (800) 227-2345, or visiting the organization's website at Cancer.org.

LIMIT ALCOHOL

Numerous scientific studies have proven low to moderate consumption of alcoholic beverages does not pose significant health risks and may, in fact, promote health. For men, that means no more than two drinks per day; women should limit themselves to a single drink daily. A drink is 12 ounces of regular beer, five ounces of wine, or 1.5 ounces of 80-proof distilled spirits. For more information, check out the CDC's online guide to alcohol and public health at CDC.gov/alcohol.

MAINTAIN A HEALTHY WEIGHT

One in three Americans is clinically obese, according to the Centers for Disease Control and Prevention. Another one-third are overweight. Those added pounds greatly raise the risk of inviting the nation's biggest killers into your life — heart disease, cancer, and diabetes — and take a huge toll on the nation's overall health and pocketbooks. In fact, obesity-related conditions are projected to cost nearly $550 billion over the next 20 years. You can take charge to control your weight by resolving to eat a healthy diet and exercising regularly. Not sure if you're overweight? Check out the National Institutes of Health's body mass index (BMI) calculator to see if you weight too much for your height at NHLBI.NIH.gov.

EAT HEALTHY

If you're trying to shed a few pounds or maintain a healthy weight, you don't need to go in for a fad diet, greatly restrict what you eat, or consider diet pills or weight-loss surgery (options intended largely for obese individuals who haven't had success with less-drastic approaches). Simply watch your portion sizes and eat more fruits, vegetables, nuts, legumes, lean protein (such as fish), and whole grains instead of fatty fried foods or animal products. Aim to eat at least 2.5 cups of nutrient-rich fruits and veggies each day. Choose whole-grain rice, breads, pastas, and cereal instead of processed (refined) grains. Limit the amount of processed meats you eat, and go for smaller portions of lean protein sources, such as skinless chicken, fish, legumes (beans and peas) and lower-fat meats (loin or round cuts). Choose foods low in saturated fat, trans fat, cholesterol, sodium, and added sugar and sweeteners (including sweetened beverages). Think of the food you eat as medicine and recognize what you put in your mouth can either increase or reduce your risk of developing heart disease, cancer, diabetes, and other obesity-related conditions. A good place to help you start developing a healthier diet: The US Department of Agriculture's website at ChooseMyPlate.gov.

GET MOVING

Gyms and health clubs, including many chains catering to older Americans, are becoming nearly as common as fast-food joints in the United States, and that's probably a healthy trend. But you don't need to join an expensive fitness center to meet federal health recommendations for physical exercise. Even a little bit of physical activity is better than none. But you should aim to get at least 150 minutes of moderate-intensity or 75 minutes of vigorous intensity activity each week (or a combination). Moderate-intensity activities include walking briskly (three miles per hour or faster, but not race-walking), water aerobics, bicycling slower than 10 miles per hour, tennis (doubles), ballroom dancing, and gardening. According to the CDC, vigorous-intensity activities include race-walking, jogging, running, swimming laps, tennis (singles), aerobic dancing, bicycling 10 miles per hour or faster, jumping rope, heavy gardening (continuous digging or hoeing), and hiking uphill or with a heavy backpack. It's best to spread your activities out through the week, getting between 20 and 30 minutes almost every day. And be sure to limit the time you spend sitting, which, for prolonged periods, can raise your risk of heart disease, diabetes, and certain cancers nearly as much as smoking.

THE "GOLDILOCKS EFFECT" FOR HEART RATE

How can you tell if you're exercising hard enough, but not putting too much stress on your heart and body? In general, you want to raise your heart rate (the number of times your heart beats per minute) to between 50 percent and 85 percent of its maximum capacity and maintain that level for at least 20 minutes. (Your maximum heart rate is about 220 minus your age). You can calculate your heart rate by counting beats while checking a stopwatch or performing what the CDC refers to as the "talk test" — pushing yourself hard enough to be able to have a conversation as you're

TABLE 12-1: HEART RATES PER AGE

Age	Target HR Zone 50-85%	Average Maximum Heart Rate, 100%
20 years	100-170 beats per minute	200 beats per minute
30 years	95-162 beats per minute	190 beats per minute
35 years	93-157 beats per minute	185 beats per minute
40 years	90-153 beats per minute	180 beats per minute
45 years	88-149 beats per minute	175 beats per minute
50 years	85-145 beats per minute	170 beats per minute
55 years	83-140 beats per minute	165 beats per minute
60 years	80-136 beats per minute	160 beats per minute
65 years	78-132 beats per minute	155 beats per minute
70 years	75-128 beats per minute	150 beats per minute

Source: American Heart Association, Target Heart Rates, http://www.heart.org

exercising, but not so hard that you can't sing a song without feeling breathless. As a rule of thumb, you're doing moderate-intensity activity if you can talk, but not sing, during the activity. If you're doing vigorous-intensity activity, you will not be able to say more than a few words without pausing for a breath.

As a reference guide, the Table 12-1 shows estimated target average heart rates for different ages.

You can also check out the American Heart Association's online heart-rate calculator at Heart.org/HEARTORG/GettingHealthy/PhysicalActivity/Target-Heart-Rates_UCM_434341_Article.jsp.

GET REGULAR PHYSICAL EXAMS

Find a doctor and be sure to seek a wellness examination at least once a year. You take your car for regular tune-ups and oil changes to keep it running in tip-top shape; why wouldn't you do the same for your body and mind? A regular exam can help establish a baseline health level and allow you to begin heart-healthy and cancer-related screenings — including those for blood pressure, cholesterol, glucose, pulse, and body mass index. A regular doctor can also help you identify health risks tied to your genetics and family background.

DO SOMETHING TO MANAGE STRESS AND GET A GOOD NIGHT'S SLEEP

Many health experts believe death certificates will one day identify a leading cause of mortality as "stress." A growing body of research has tied long-term, chronic stress to a variety of health conditions, including increased heart rate and blood pressure, which can damage the heart; lowered immune system function, which can increase the risks of cancer, diabetes; and higher levels of anxiety and depression that can boost the odds of mental-health conditions, dementia, and Alzheimer's disease later in life. Poor sleep habits can also put you at risk for the nation's biggest killers. Take steps to manage stress and any sleep problems you may have as if your life depended on it (which it just may). One in five adults has at least mild sleep apnea, which can contribute to high blood pressure, heart disease, and stroke. Learn and practice stress-management techniques (including yoga, meditation, or simply engaging in a quiet activity you enjoy for at least a few minutes every day). Aim to get between seven and nine hours of sleep each night and seek help if you struggle to fall asleep and stay asleep because of insomnia, sleep apnea, or other conditions that keep you awake at night.

Screening Recommendations: As You Age

OK, so now you know the basic guidelines for aging gracefully — and healthfully. And let's presume you managed to cruise through your 20s and 30s without a significant health problem. Good for you! You must be doing something right. Chances are you followed at least some of the recommended guidelines for health and wellness, based on your family history and individual risk factors, and have tried to at least pay some attention to your diet and fitness.

But once you hit your 40s, you can't take your health for granted and bank on the vitality of your younger years to keep you healthy. It's critically important to pay more attention to health-screening guidelines for your age group. For instance, cancer-related check-ups should be part of your regular health exams and might include screening for cancers of the thyroid, mouth, skin, lymph nodes, testicles, or ovaries.

Now's also the time to review with your doctor what you can, and should, be doing to reduce your risks for cardiovascular disease, diabetes, and psychological conditions — all of which increase with advancing age.

To help you get started, here is a list of tests for certain cancers that are recommended as you enter your 40s and beyond:

MEN: 40 AND OLDER

Colon Cancer Testing

You should determine now if you are at higher risk for colon cancer because of family history or other factors. If you are at increased risk, talk to your doctor about what testing is right for you and when it should begin. If not, no test is needed at this age.

Prostate Cancer Testing

If prostate cancer runs in your family or you face a higher risk for other reasons, you should

ABOUT PSA TESTS

Although there has been much debate over the effectiveness of prostate-specific antigen (PSA) tests, many doctors recommend men have a PSA test by their mid-40s to at least establish a baseline to which future results can be compared. A single PSA test may not be a useful gauge of a man's prostate cancer risk, but a trendline dating back several years or even decades can help your doctor take the best care of you, should your PSA rise as you grow older.

talk to your doctor about what tests are appropriate for you and when they should begin. This includes African-Americans and men with close family members (father, brother, son) who have had prostate cancer. You should also know that young men diagnosed with prostate cancer — before age 65 — face substantially higher risks. Two of the most common prostate tests are the digital rectal exam, during which a doctor feels for abnormalities, and the PSA test — short for prostate-specific antigen, a biomarker detected by a blood test that can indicate the presence of cancer or other prostate problems. Any irregularity turned up by a DRE or PSA test can be followed up with a biopsy to check for cancerous tissue.

WOMEN: 40 AND OLDER

Breast Cancer Testing

All women in their 40s should have an annual breast exam, performed by your doctor or nurse. You should also learn to do a self-exam and report any lumps or breast changes to your doctor. Although mammograms — breast X-rays — are not as reliable in detecting cancer in healthy women before 50, many authorities — including the American Cancer Society — recommend having one every year beginning at age 40. If you are at higher risk for breast cancer than most women because of lifestyle factors or a family history of breast cancer, ask a healthcare professional about additional tests.

Cervical Cancer Testing

Beginning at age 40, you should have a Pap test and HPV test every five years or a Pap test alone every three years. This is true even if you have been vaccinated against HPV, the virus known to cause cervical cancer. If you have had a hysterectomy and had your uterus and cervix removed, there is no reason for such testing.

Colon Cancer Testing

Take steps to determine now if you are at higher risk for colon cancer because of family history or other factors. If you are at increased risk, talk to your doctor about what testing is right for you and when it should begin. If not, no test is needed at this age.

BOTH SEXES: 40 AND OLDER
Watch your weight

Your metabolism starts to slow in your 40s, which increases the odds of packing on the pounds, stressing your heart and raising the risk of developing Type 2 diabetes. Now's the age to establish a regular fitness routine, if you haven't already, and follow a heart-healthy diet.

Check your blood sugar levels

By age 40-45, you should be having regular checks of your heart rate, blood pressure, and fasting blood glucose, to identify any problems and establish a baseline for future comparison tests. Such checks should be done earlier if you are overweight, diabetic, or at risk for heart disease.

MEN: 50 TO 65
Colon Cancer Testing

It may not be something you look forward to as you celebrate your 50th birthday, but this is the year when you should have your first colonoscopy — with a follow-up every five years (or fewer, if you are at risk for colon cancer). There are several other colon-cancer screening options, so talk with your doctor about which tests are best for you and how frequently tests should be done.

Prostate Cancer Testing

Beginning at age 50, you should consult your doctor about the uncertainties, risks, and potential benefits of yearly PSA testing and other screening for prostate cancer to decide the best course of action.

WOMEN: 50 TO 65
Breast Cancer Screening

By age 50, women should have an annual mammogram. If you are at higher risk for breast cancer than most women because of your lifestyle or family history, consult a healthcare professional about additional options, including available genetic tests that can determine if you carry defective genes — known as BRCA1 and BRCA2 — that significantly increase the odds you could develop breast cancer.

A note about breast cancer genes: Some women who carry such genetic mutations, most notably actress Angelina Jolie, have chosen to have preventive mastectomies to lower their risks. But other, less drastic options can also make a difference and reduce your odds of being diagnosed with cancer, including increased medical vigilance and lifestyle changes that can compensate for your genetic predisposition toward the disease. It's important to note that genes are not destiny; just because your genetic makeup increases the likelihood you may develop cancer doesn't mean you actually will. Cancer typically results from a combination of factors, including genetics and lifestyle. As cancer specialists like to say "Genetics loads the gun, lifestyle pulls the trigger." As a result, getting tested for breast cancer genes can help you adjust your lifestyle to cut the odds that you'll develop cancer — by eating a healthy diet, exercising regularly and engaging in other behaviors known to stave off the disease — even if your family heritage puts you at greater risk.

Cervical Cancer Testing
Continue having a Pap test and HPV test every five years or a Pap test alone every three years, and follow your doctors' guidance on how best to reduce your risks.

Colon Cancer Testing
As with men, women should have their first colonoscopy at age 50 and a follow-up every three to five years thereafter, depending on your particular risk factors. You should also explore other screening options with your doctor.

BOTH SEXES: 50 TO 65
Learn Stroke, Heart Attack Symptoms
Now is the time to learn the warning signs of a heart attack (chest pain, weakness, shortness of breath, sweating, nausea) and stroke (face drooping, arm weakness, difficulty speaking). It's also important to recognize that heart attack symptoms in women can be very different than what men experience.

The crushing chest pain most commonly associated with cardiac arrest in men is not as common in women, who typically experience less dramatic symptoms, such as shortness of breath, pressure or pain in the lower chest or upper abdomen, dizziness, lightheadedness, nausea/vomiting, fainting, upper back pressure, or fatigue. That's one reason many women — and the doctors who treat them — may not take such symptoms as seriously or treat them as aggressively as in men. But such misconceptions can be deadly. Heart disease is the number one killer of women and men, in the United States, causing more deaths than all cancers combined (including breast and prostate cancer).

According to the American Heart Association, a heart attack occurs in the US about every 34 seconds, causing a stoppage of blood flow that brings oxygen to the heart muscle, usually because of a buildup of fat, cholesterol or other substances in blood vessels.

MEN AND WOMEN: OVER 65

Once you hit your mid-60s, the risk of being diagnosed with cancer and heart disease increases significantly. As a result you should begin talking with your doctor about annual or regular screening for virtually all types of cardiovascular disease and cancer: thyroid, mouth, skin, lymph nodes, testicles, ovaries, colon, prostate, breast.

It's important to talk to your doctor about the uncertainties, risks, and benefits of various types of testing. The good news: Most disease-prevention testing is covered under Medicare, including mammograms, colonoscopies, diabetes tests, flu shots, mental health, and cardiovascular screenings — and will cost you nothing.

Realize that with advancing age, your blood pressure, cholesterol, and other heart-related vital statistics tend to rise. That's why it's important to keep a close watch on your numbers and manage any health conditions that arise.

Beyond the "Big C"

Ask most Americans to identify the biggest cause of death in the United States and most are likely to say cancer. Most would be wrong. In fact, cardiovascular disease kills far more Americans than cancer.

According to the Centers for Disease Control and Prevention, heart disease is the leading cause of death in the United States (killing 597,689 Americans every year), followed by cancer (574,743 deaths), chronic lower respiratory diseases (138,080), stroke (129,476), accidents (120,859), Alzheimer's disease-related complications (83,494), diabetes (69,071), nephritis, nephrotic syndrome, and nephrosis (50,476), influenza and pneumonia (50,097), and suicide (38,364).

The American Heart Association puts those figures into perspective by noting that heart and vascular conditions kill 2,150 people each day — about one death every 40 seconds — which adds up to nearly a third of all causes of death.

But as startling as such statistics are, perhaps what is most surprising is the fact that the majority of Americans underestimate the impact of heart disease on health. This is particularly true when it comes to breast cancer, which tends to get more attention than heart disease, as a woman's health issue. One reason: misconceptions about cardiovascular risks among women — and even some doctors who treat them — are partly to blame.

A recent study published in *Global Heart* (the journal of the World Heart Federation) by researchers from Ohio State University found that awareness of women's risks of developing coronary artery disease (CAD) has increased over the past decade, but men are still more aggressively treated at the first signs of the heart-related condition.

The researchers noted CAD kills as many women as men each year, but doctors are less likely to recommend preventive measures for women, compared to men at risk — such as lowering cholesterol, taking aspirin, or making lifestyle changes in their dietary and exercise habits. One reason: It is still largely considered a "man's disease" by many women and doctors who should know better, according to lead researchers Martha Gulati, MD, and Kavita Sharma, MD.

"One in three women get heart disease; one in two get heart disease or stroke, and one in eight get breast cancer," says Dr. Gulati. "One in four women dies from heart disease and one in 30 women dies from breast cancer. Heart disease is the number one killer of women. Lack of awareness is a [factor]."

According to the study, cardiovascular diseases are the leading cause of death for men and women worldwide, killing 8.6 million women alone each year. That's one-third of all deaths in women.

According to the American Heart Association, cardiovascular disease — including heart disease, high blood pressure, and stroke — kills more women in the US each year than next seven causes of death combined. More women die from CAD than of all cancers (including breast cancer, which kills about 40,000 women annually), respiratory conditions, Alzheimer's disease, and accidents. Women are also more likely than men to die of a heart attack and twice as likely to have a second heart attack in the six years following the first.

The new study did note the overall death rate from heart disease in the US has dropped by 30 percent since 1998. But rates among women under 55 years old are still rising, with women under 50 who have a heart attack twice as likely as men to die. What's more, 42 percent of women who have heart attacks die within a year, compared to 24 percent of men.

Dr. Gulati, a cardiologist at Ohio State and author of the book *Saving Women's Hearts: How You Can Prevent and Reverse Heart Disease With Natural and Conventional Strategies*, notes symptoms of heart disease in women are often different from men.

For instance, the dramatic, crushing chest pain men feel when a heart attack strikes is not as common in women, who are more likely to feel less alarming arm pain and experience shortness of breath. Many women may merely feel sick to their stomach or like they have the flu. Women may also feel anxiety, dizziness, fatigue, a dull ache in their left arm, jaw, chest, or back instead of the more severe painful symptoms men experience.

The new research highlights other differences between men's and women's heart risks:

Obesity (tied to lack of exercise and unhealthy diets) increases the risk of CAD by 64 percent in women but only 46 percent in men.

CT scans and other imaging techniques show that women have narrower coronary arteries than do men, which may account for the greater risks women face.

Women with an immediate family member who has had CAD face greater risks than men.

Diabetes raises a woman's CAD risk by three to seven times, while for men it is two to three times.

The researchers said awareness of the impact of CAD on women is growing, but is still low. In 1997, for instance, only 30 percent of American women surveyed were aware that the leading cause of death in women is heart disease. By 2009, that level of awareness had grown to 54 percent. But that figure still indicates many women mistakenly believe breast cancer is a bigger threat to their lives than heart disease. In addition, fewer than one in five physicians recognize that more women than men die each year from CAD.

"I think [the public awareness campaign] about breast cancer screening is a huge success," Dr. Gulati says. "We have not done the same yet for heart disease.

"[Resolving the issue] is going to take increasing women's awareness, increasing physician awareness, teaching this within nursing and medical schools, and making cardiac screening an essential part of primary care . . . The big issue lies in the fact right now that if a woman has a heart attack she is less likely to get the same treatment as a man. That needs to change."

Of course, heart disease, is not exclusively a women's health issue. But the Ohio State research highlights the need for men and women alike to be aware of the importance of healthy lifestyle choices. Follow the diet and exercise tips recommended in this chapter, being sure to choose activities (along with exercise) that will reduce stress, such as meditation or a relaxing pastime.

The bottom line, says Alan S. Go, MD, chief of the Cardiovascular and Metabolic Conditions Section of the Kaiser Permanente Northern California Division of Research in Oakland: "Americans need to move a lot more, eat healthier and less, and manage risk factors as soon as they develop. If not, we'll quickly lose the momentum we've gained in reducing heart attack and stroke rates and improving survival over the last few decades."

Minding Your Mental Health

As health statistics go, the numbers are simply staggering:

- **5 million:** Americans with Alzheimer's and other forms of dementia (44 million worldwide), with a new US diagnosis made every 68 seconds

- **13.8 million:** Projected US cases of dementia by 2050 (135 million worldwide)

- **1 in 3:** US seniors who die with dementia today

- **$203 billion:** Cost for Alzheimer's care in the United States today ($600 billion worldwide) — expenditures that are projected to increase fivefold over the next 40 years

These latest facts and figures from the Alzheimer's Association and Alzheimer's Disease International underscore what many health experts believe is a global epidemic that is growing worse by the day.

"If we look into the future the numbers of elderly people will rise dramatically," noted ADI's Executive Director Marc Wortmann. "It's vital that the World Health Organization makes dementia a priority, so the world is ready to face this condition."

Now for the good news: A growing body of research suggests many of the things you can do to maintain a healthy body also benefit the brain and reduce the risk of the mind-wasting, age-related disorder — from exercise to diet to healthy lifestyle habits. In addition, a number of studies support the use-it-or-lose-it approach to mental health, providing strong evidence that an active mind and body can stave off dementia and Alzheimer's.

"What the research shows is that following a healthy lifestyle confers surprisingly large benefits to [mental] health," noted Peter Elwood, a Cardiff University School of Medicine health specialist who recently published a 35-year study showing the five lifestyle behaviors that most significantly reduce the risk of age-related cognitive decline. Practicing these behaviors may be more beneficial than medical treatments or other preventive measures.

The findings, based on an analysis of the medical charts of 2,235 men from 1979 to 2004, in Caerphilly, Wales, UK, tied the following five healthy behaviors to a lower risk for Alzheimer's: regular exercise, not smoking, keeping a low bodyweight, following a healthy diet, and having a low alcohol intake.

"The size of reduction in the instance of disease owing to these simple healthy steps has really amazed us and is of enormous importance in an aging population," said Elwood, whose research was published in the Public Library of Science journal *PLOS One*.

Elwood's work isn't the only scientific research to support the idea of a mind-body connection when it comes to physical and mental health. Here's a breakdown of five scientifically proven ways to protect yourself against Alzheimer's and dementia.

5 Rules to Live By

NO 1: EXERCISE

Regular aerobic activity — running, brisk walking, swimming, biking — boosts blood flow and the flood of oxygen to the brain and other key organs of the body. Studies have shown people who engage in such activity are far more likely to stay mentally sharp as they age.

Sports scientists at the Center for Brain Health at the University of Texas at Dallas have found, for instance, that getting as little as one hour of aerobic exercise three times a week can boost memory and brain function. The federally funded UT study, published in the journal *Frontiers in Aging Neuroscience*, tracked a group of sedentary adults, ages 57-75, who engaged in supervised exercise on a stationary bike or treadmill for one hour, three times a week for 12 weeks.

Tests of the participants' cognition, resting cerebral blood flow, and cardiovascular fitness showed significant improvements in memory and had a greater increase in brain blood flow to the hippocampus, the key brain region affected by Alzheimer's disease, as measured by brain scans.

"Science has shown that aging decreases mental efficiency and memory decline is the number one cognitive complaint of older adults," said lead researcher Sandra Bond Chapman, director of the Center for BrainHealth. "This research shows the tremendous benefit of aerobic exercise on a person's memory and demonstrates that aerobic exercise can reduce both the biological and cognitive consequences of aging."

Chapman added that exercise "may be one of the most beneficial and cost-effective therapies widely available to everyone to elevate memory performance. These findings should motivate adults of all ages to start exercising aerobically."

Other recent studies have reinforced Chapman's findings:

- Scientists with the National Institute on Aging have found being in good physical shape helps preserve people's thinking and memory skills. In research involving 1,400 people, investigators found 80-year-olds who are twice as fit as their peers made about 25 percent fewer errors on a test of memory and concentration. "This study shows that your cardiovascular fitness at one point in time can predict how well your memory may function in the future," said Carrington Wendell, a researcher with institute who led the 2013 study.

- British researchers who tracked 3,500 people found those who engaged in regular physical activity throughout their lives were seven times less likely to suffer dementia and other major illnesses late in life. The 2013 study, published in the *British Journal of Sports Medicine*, found exercise was the biggest factor in what they termed "healthy aging" in the men and women, whose average age was 64. Healthy aging is defined as the absence of major disease and disability, good mental health, the preservation of cognitive abilities, and the ability to maintain social connections/activities.

- Harvard Medical School research has demonstrated that strength training — lifting weights or doing other weight-bearing or resistance exercises — a few times a week is also critical to maintaining a sharp mental edge and muscle mass after age 50. The average 30-year-old will lose about a quarter of his or her muscle strength by age 70 and half of it by age 90, notes Dr. Robert Schreiber, Harvard Medical instructor.

FYI: For more information on exercise recommendations, visit the US Department of Health and Human Service's guide to physical activity at Health.gov/paguidelines/.

NO. 2: WEIGHT CONTROL

People who are overweight (with a BMI between 25 and 30) are twice as likely to develop Alzheimer's, and those who are considered clinically obese face a threefold increased risk. The reason: Packing on extra pounds leads to fat deposits in the brain and narrowed blood vessels, restricting their ability to deliver fuel and oxygen. Over time, brain cells die and the brain shrinks, causing memory loss, confusion, and other cognitive problems that make it difficult to carry out everyday tasks and live independently.

The remedy: Maintain a healthy weight by eating a sensible diet that is low in fat, fried foods, sugar, and refined flour and high in nutrient-rich fruits and vegetables, whole grains, legumes, fish, and other lean protein sources, as previously referenced. Some evidence also shows that green, leafy, cruciferous vegetables, foods high in omega-3 fatty acids (such as oily fish), and nuts (which have high levels of vitamin E) — all staples of the Mediterranean diet — may be protective against Alzheimer's.

Researchers with the Westmead Millennium Institute for Medical Research at the University of Sydney in New South Wales,

Australia, have found older adults who follow recommended dietary guidelines have a higher quality of life and less trouble taking care of themselves.

The study, reported in the *Journal of the Academy of Nutrition and Dietetics*, is based on an analysis of the diets and mental-health status of 1,305 men and women aged 55 and over. On average, participants with the healthiest diets reported a better quality of life, and more robust physical and mental-health functioning. Those with the highest-rated diets were also half as likely to be impaired when it came to how well they could perform basic and instrumental activities of daily living — such as eating, dressing, and grooming without assistance, as well as shopping, using a telephone, handling money, and traveling beyond walking distance.

"Higher diet quality was prospectively associated with better quality of life and functional ability," the researchers concluded.

Eating a healthy diet and controlling your weight will also help hold down levels of cholesterol and high blood pressure — all of which are strong risk factors for Alzheimer's, in part because they boost the odds of developing Type 2 diabetes and heart disease (which affect brain function and may contribute to the development or severity of dementia).

FYI: For help in figuring out how to improve your diet, check out the US Department of Agriculture's "MyPlate" guide — ChooseMyPlate.gov — for tips and suggestions.

NO. 3: MENTAL CHALLENGES

Use it or lose it. In the most simple terms, that may be your best strategy for maintaining a sharp mental edge as you age. Not long ago, neurologists believed brain cells stopped forming and developing in adulthood, but new research on the brain has overturned those earlier theories. In fact, new information and experiences drive important changes and developments in the brain's neural pathways, leading to new connections and even generating new brain cells at every age.

Like the muscles of your body, you need to exercise your brain — challenging yourself mentally with new experiences — to keep it in tip-top shape. For the nation's baby boomers, that means retirement can't be a period of dialing down and easing back, but must be a passage in life that involves new activities, learning experiences, and engagement with disciplines of the mind.

In fact, the more you want to use your brain, the more likely you are to stay sharp as you age, according to recent findings by a team of Canadian researchers from Concordia University's Department of Psychology.

This study, published in the October 2013 issue of *Journals of Gerontology: Psychological Sciences*, was based on an analysis of information gathered from 333 recent retirees — with an average age of 59 — who underwent assessments of cognition, motivation, and activities once a year. The researchers reached three major conclusions about factors that can help forecast cognitive ability later in life:

- The more a person seeks out and enjoys cognitively demanding activities, the less likely he or she is to experience age-related cognitive decline.

- Engaging in a variety of different mentally-challenging activities — reading, learning new tasks, doing crossword puzzles — can help boost brainpower at any age.

- People who have even mild depression are more likely to show a decline in brainpower, particularly post-retirement, when they may not be as engaged or challenged in their everyday lives.

Lead researcher Larry Baer said the findings have particular significance for baby boomers at or nearing retirement age.

"Retirement usually occurs right around the time when normal age-related declines in cognitive function come to the fore," said Baer, in comments that accompanied the study's release. "So it is important to understand what is happening to brainpower during this period and to identify risk factors for mental decline, as well as factors that will help protect against it."

Challenging your mind doesn't have to involve crossword puzzles or becoming a bookworm. Try picking up a musical instrument, learning a new language, or traveling to a place you've never been before.

Researchers at the University of St. Andrews in Scotland have demonstrated that people who practice playing musical instruments have sharper brains, perhaps because they have to pick up mistakes in their performance and fix them more quickly than other people — a learned skill that can apply to a range of non-musical settings.

Writing about their work in the journal *Neuropsychologia,* psychologist Ines Jentzsch and colleagues said the findings strongly suggest playing music may help ward off age-related mental declines. The findings echoed a 2013 review of 400 research papers on the neurochemistry of music that found playing and even listening to music benefits mental and physical health by boosting the immune system and easing stress. The report, published in *Trends in Cognitive Sciences,* was funded by the Social Sciences and Humanities Research Council and the Natural Sciences and Engineering Research Council (NSERC).

And while the greatest affects are seen in those who play and practice music more frequently, you don't have to become a professional to benefit.

"Our study shows that even moderate levels of musical activity can benefit brain functioning," said Jentzsch, who is affiliated with St. Andrews' School of Psychology and Neuroscience and a pianist herself. "The research suggests that musical activity could be used as an effective intervention to slow, stop, or even reverse age- or illness-related decline in mental functioning.

She added that the benefits are evident at any age, indicating "it's never too late" to pick up a musical instrument and learn to play. "Musical activity cannot only immensely enrich our lives, but the associated benefits for our physical and mental functioning could be even more far-reaching than proposed in our and previous research," she said.

An international team of scientists has found that learning a second language can also help ward off dementia, and may even help build brainpower in individuals who have already been diagnosed with Alzheimer's. The 2013 study, carried out by researchers from the University of Edinburgh and Nizam's Institute of Medical Sciences in Hyderabad in India, examined almost 650 dementia patients and assessed when each one had been diagnosed with the condition.

The findings, published in the medical journal *Neurology,* showed those who spoke two or more languages experienced a later onset (by five or more years) of Alzheimer's disease, vascular dementia, and frontotemporal dementia than those who spoke only one tongue.

The tendency held true regardless of a person's education, gender, and occupation. The reasons are unclear, but mental-health experts suspect that bilingual switching between different sounds, words, concepts, grammatical structures, and social norms constitutes a form of natural brain training, the brain-boosting, mental workout we get from learning or practicing music or math skills.

Bilingualism may also build what neurologists refer to as "brain reserve" — the ability of the brain to keep functioning normally despite significant disease or injury. Past studies have shown education, higher occupational status, and regular engagement in higher-order thinking activities can all boost brain reserve, which can delay the onset of dementia and lessen its severity.

The international team that conducted the latest study said that speaking two languages may also contribute to cognitive reserve.

"These findings suggest that bilingualism might have a stronger influence on dementia than any currently available drugs," said Thomas Bak, of the University of Edinburgh's School of Philosophy, Psychology, and Language Sciences. "This makes the study of the relationship between bilingualism and cognition one of our highest priorities."

NO. 4: SOCIAL INTERACTIONS

Staying connected with family and friends doesn't just make you more social and outgoing, it may also keep you mentally sharper as the years roll by. Studies have shown people with larger social networks tend to experience less mental decline — as they age than seniors who have much less interaction — even when both groups of individuals have the same levels of plaques in the brain associated with Alzheimer's.

While researchers can't say precisely why this is so, many psychologists suspect social interaction stimulates the brain to make new connections that help stave off mental decline and even dementia — something not seen in more withdrawn and isolated people.

Memory and aging specialists with Chicago's Rush University Medical Center have demonstrated, for instance, that seniors who spend lots of time with friends and relatives tend to have fewer symptoms of dementia than isolated older individuals. The Rush study, published in *The Lancet Neurology* medical journal, is based on analysis of nearly 90 people who were monitored from the time they were in their early 80s until death.

Every year, participants were screened for Alzheimer's and took 21 tests of mental skills including memory and reading. They also reported how many close friends and relatives they visited with every month.

After the participants died, autopsies were performed to determine the amount of plaques in their brains — features linked to Alzheimer's.

The results clearly showed that seniors with larger social networks generally scored higher on their mental and memory tests, even if they were later found to have more severe amounts of brain plaque.

"These results were unchanged after [accounting] for cognitive, physical, and social activities, depressive symptoms, or number of chronic diseases," the researchers concluded.

The take-home message is obvious: Stay connected with friends and relatives, no matter what age you are. Join a club with people who share your interests. Volunteer your time to a worthy cause. Get active with a political organization. Play a team sport. Indulge in a hobby that puts you in contact with other like-minded folks. Think about taking an adult-education class or participate in any activity that allows you to connect with others who share your passion for life and social interaction.

For more ideas on building and expanding your social network, visit AARP.org.

NO. 5: CUT DOWN ON STRESS

You already know stress is bad for your heart. But did you know high levels of stress — beginning in midlife — can set off a cascade of biochemical processes in the brain that can heighten the risk of dementia later in life?

Research published in the online medical journal, *BMJ Open*, found women who have a hard time coping with the stresses of common life events experience long-lasting physiological changes in the brain that predispose them to Alzheimer's and other forms of dementia.

To reach their conclusions, mental-health experts from Gothenburg University in Sweden tracked the mental health and well-being of 800 Swedish women for nearly 40 years, beginning 1968. The women, who were born between 1914 and 1930, underwent a battery of neuropsychiatric tests and examinations in 1968, and then again in 1974, 1980, 1992, 2000, and 2005. Researchers quizzed the women about the psychological impact of 18 common stressors, such as divorce, widowhood, serious illness, death of a child, mental illness or alcoholism in a close family member, personal or partner's unemployment, and poor social support.

Over the course of the study, more than half of the women died (at the average age of 79), one in five (153) developed dementia, and one in eight (104) were diagnosed with Alzheimer's disease.

When the researchers cross-checked the women's medical charts and survey information, they found those with a high number of stressful life events had a 36 percent heightened risk of developing Alzheimer's disease and or other forms of dementia. The findings held true even after taking account of factors likely to influence the results, including a family history of mental health problems.

They concluded: "Stress may cause a number of physiological reactions in the central nervous, endocrine, immune and cardiovascular systems."

Other studies have also linked stress to structural and functional damage to the brain and inflammation. Stress hormones triggered by difficult life events are also known to remain at high levels many years after some people experience a traumatic event, causing serious harm to the immune system and key organs of the body.

Conversely, a number of recent scientific studies have proven what Eastern mystics have known for centuries: Meditation and other stress-reduction techniques — including yoga, exercise, or simply spending quiet time alone for a few minutes each day — are good for the mind as well as the body. More to the point: A number of research efforts have demonstrated beyond a shadow of doubt that cutting stress can boost the immune system and produce measurable changes in the brain that reduce the risk of developing Alzheimer's and dementia.

A recent federally funded study by researchers at Beth Israel Deaconess Medical Center in Boston found, for instance, that positive changes in the brain are noticeable after just two months of practicing stress-reduction techniques for as little as 15 to 30 minutes each day. The 2013 study, funded by the National Institutes of

Health and published in the journal *Neuroscience Letters*, suggests that positive changes appear to stave off or slow the progression of Alzheimer's disease and dementia.

"We know that approximately 50 percent of people diagnosed with mild cognitive impairment — the intermediate stage between the expected declines of normal aging and the more serious cognitive deterioration associated with dementia — may develop dementia within five years," said Rebecca Erwin Wells, MD, who conducted her research as a fellow in Integrative Medicine at Beth Israel and Harvard Medical School. "And unfortunately, we know there are currently no FDA-approved medications that can stop that progression.

"We also know that as people age, there's a high correlation between perceived stress and Alzheimer's disease, so we wanted to know if stress reduction through meditation might improve cognitive reserve."

For the study, Dr. Wells and her colleagues evaluated the effects of yoga and meditation classes on 14 adults, between 55 and 90 years old, who were diagnosed with mild cognitive impairment. All participants underwent a functional MRI (fMRI) at the beginning and end of the study to track changes in the areas of the brain related to memory, learning, and emotions — the regions that tend to atrophy as Alzheimer's disease progresses.

Participants were divided into two groups: One attended meditation and yoga classes for two hours each week for eight weeks, participated in a day-long mindfulness retreat, and were encouraged to continue their practice at home for 15 to 30 minutes per day. The other did not engage in any of the stress-reduction techniques.

The results of the study showed that the meditating group had significantly improved brain function and less atrophy than those participants who did not engage in meditation or yoga.

"This is a small study and more research is needed to further investigate these results, but we're very excited about these findings because they suggest that [stress-reduction practices] may [improve function] in the same areas of the brain most affected by Alzheimer's disease," Dr. Wells said.

"If [meditating] can help delay the symptoms of cognitive decline even a little bit, it can contribute to improved quality of life for many of these patients."

FYI: To learn more about the benefits and practice of stress-reduction techniques, visit the NIH Center for Complementary and Alternative Medicine at NCCAM.NIH.gov/health/providers/digest/relaxation.htm.

Beware of Bogus Cancer Cures

You see the ads every day: Online, on television, and on the pages of every newspaper in the country, claims of new products offer miracle cures for everything from cancer to AIDS, heart disease, diabetes, Alzheimer's, and even erectile dysfunction.

The truth is that such "cures" are bogus, but with an expanding proportion of the nation growing older and being diagnosed with chronic conditions, the appeal of such marketing schemes is irresistible to many. Plus, an ample body of research suggests many seniors are particularly vulnerable to such scams for reasons that have to do as much with brain chemistry as a natural instinct to trust what they read and hear to be true, until proven otherwise.

That combination allows scam artists to prey upon individuals who are most vulnerable.

The Federal Drug Administration lists bogus, "crackpot cures" on its website, www.FDA.gov/forconsumers/protectyourself/healthfraud/default.htm, warning consumers to avoid tablets, creams, teas, black salves, and tonics known to be scams.

"Anyone who suffers from cancer, or knows someone who does, understands the fear and desperation that can set in," says Gary Coody, the National Health Fraud Coordinator and a Consumer Safety Officer with the FDA's Office of Regulatory Affairs. "There can be a great temptation to jump at anything that appears to offer a chance for a cure."

It's important to understand that medicinal products and devices intended to treat cancer and other conditions must gain FDA approval before they are marketed. The agency's review process helps ensure that these products are safe and effective.

Nevertheless, it's always possible to find someone or some company hawking bogus, non-FDA-approved treatments.

"They're frequently offered as natural treatments and 'dietary supplements,' " says Coody. "Advertisements and other promotional materials touting bogus cancer 'cures' have probably been around as long as the printing press. However, the Internet has compounded the problem by providing the peddlers of these often dangerous products a whole new outlet."

At best, such bogus treatments are a waste of money. But at worst they may prevent some people from seeking more effective therapies in a timely manner or even cause harm because they may contain toxic ingredients or active agents that interfere with prescription medications.

To protect yourself, the FDA recommends avoiding products marketed with the following phrases that should be red flags:

- Treats all forms of cancer

- Shrinks malignant tumors

- Non-toxic

- Doesn't make you sick

- Avoid painful surgery, radiotherapy, chemotherapy, or other conventional treatments

Health experts also recommend being wary about products accompanied by "personal testimonies" by individuals who claim the product works (who are often paid actors), those offering a money-back guarantee, or those requiring advance payments.

Other suspicious phrases, according to the American Society of Clinical Oncology, are "scientific breakthrough," "miraculous cure," "secret ingredient," or "ancient remedy." These terms may sound impressive, but advertisers can easily use them without offering proof to support their claims.

Coody adds that it's always a good idea to consult with your doctor before starting a new treatment or adding one to existing therapies. It's also important to understand the difference between fraudulent drug products and what the FDA calls "investigational drugs" undergoing clinical testing to determine if they are safe and effective for their intended uses.

"There are legal ways for patients to access investigational drugs," says Coody. "The most common way is by taking part in clinical trials. But patients can also receive investigational drugs outside of clinical trials in some cases."

It's also important to note that many supplements on the market are fake, with a recent study by Canadian researchers determining many products don't contain what's on the label. They used DNA barcoding — a type of genetic fingerprinting — to test 44 bottles of supplements sold by 12 companies in the United States and Canada. The results, published in the journal *BMC Medicine*, showed many pills did not contain the ingredients on the labels; some were diluted or contained fillers like soybean, wheat, and rice; and some contained potentially harmful substances.

For instance, bottles of echinacea, used to prevent and treat colds, were found to contain "bitter weed," a plant found in India and Australia linked to rashes and nausea; a bottle labeled as St. John's wort, a natural antidepressant, contained Alexandrian senna, an Egyptian shrub used as a laxative; and a gingko biloba supplements, promoted as memory boosters, contained unlabeled black walnut, posing a potent risk for people with nut allergies.

David Brownstein, MD, a board-certified family physician and medical director for the Center for Holistic Medicine in West Bloomfield, MI, says the new scientific analysis of supplements confirms what he has long known: Many pills labeled as healing herbs don't contain what the labels claim.

"I agree with this analysis," he said, commenting on the 2013 study. "It is the Wild, Wild West out there with supplements because there's nobody checking these things. I have been testing supplements for 20 years and finding that what's on the labels often isn't what's in the bottle."

Dr. Brownstein uses supplements in his own practice, but makes sure that he is working with trustworthy companies that verify and guarantee the products they sell.

"It's a conundrum for consumers," he says, noting the FDA does not regulate supplements like drugs so consumer information can be difficult to find on herbal supplements.

But consumers can buy products from reputable companies by taking the following precautions:

- Call the supplement manufacturers and ask for a copy of the laboratory analyses of its products.

- Work with a doctor who is well-trained in supplement use and who can perform blood tests and other medical procedures to be sure you're being treated properly.

- Check product labels for what is known as a GMP Certification, indicating the supplement manufacturer complies with a standardized set of good manufacturing practices (GMP) developed by the Natural Products Association. Under the GMP program, which is based on the FDA's Code of Regulations, certified companies agree to meet the NPA's criteria for product supplement consistency, quality, strength, and purity.

Will You Live to 100?

In the late 18th century, when the first US Census was conducted, only one in 50 Americans lived to see their 65th birthday. The concept of living to 100 was beyond most people's imagination.

But today, more than 100,000 Americans have reached the century mark and the number is rising, largely because of advances in medicine, nutrition, and health.

The latest estimates show a woman can expect to live 81 years on average; for men, the figure is 76.2 years (2010), according to the Centers for Disease Control and Prevention. Globally, the latest estimates (from 2010) show that a man's average life expectancy is about 67.5 years — up from 56.4 years in 1970. For women, it's 73.3 years — up from 61.2 years in 1970.

Japanese women have the highest life expectancy at birth in the world, at 85.9 years; for men, Iceland has the highest life expectancy, at 80.0 years. Haiti had the lowest life expectancy at birth in 2010 for both men and women (32.5 and 43.6, respectively).

So what can you do to increase your odds of celebrating your 100th birthday? Experts from a range of health specialties say the following five strategies can dramatically increase your longevity by lowering the risk of developing life-threatening chronic disease:

MOVE MORE, EAT LESS

Aim to get at least 20-30 minutes of aerobic exercise every day — more is better — and supplement it with strength-training workouts (lifting weights, resistance exercises) every other day. Eat only as many calories as you will burn in a day to maintain a healthy weight, and try to think of food as fuel for your body — the higher the nutritional value of what you eat the better.

BANISH STRESS

Stress causes your body to produce cortisol, a hormone that can hinder your immune system and create inflammation in the body tied to a host of life-threatening physical and mental health conditions. Try to think of stress reduction in the same way you think of eating, breathing, and drinking — all things you must do every day to live. Do something to relax every day — yoga, meditation, take a walk, listen to music, or just sit quietly for a few minutes.

REST UP

Aim to get about seven to nine hours of sleep every day — no more and no less. If you have trouble sleeping, invest in a good mattress (where you spend about a third of every day) and make sure your bedroom is dark, free of distractions, and comfortable. Avoid caffeine or alcohol close to bed time and be sure to manage any clinical sleep disorders you may have, such as sleep apnea, which can increase your risk of heart disease and early death.

FOLLOW YOUR BLISS

Doing what makes you happy also makes you healthy, with many studies linking a positive, upbeat outlook to a healthier, longer life. Laughing reduces your blood pressure and boosts endorphins — hormones that ease pain and increase feelings of euphoria. Make an effort to savor your time with a life companion, family, and friends — research has proven that people who are married/partnered or have close friends live longer. If you're on your own, volunteer your time with a community or nonprofit organization, but do something that makes you feel good and helps you connect with people.

LEARN NEW THINGS

Keep your brain healthy by challenging your mind to learn something new. Pick up an instrument. Learn to speak Chinese. Take up a new hobby. Sign up for a cooking class. Try using your left hand instead of your (dominant) right when doing household tasks. Whenever you learn something new, you're strengthening connections between brain cells and keeping your mind sharp — regardless of your age.

In closing, let's take a look at some of the key requirements to keep us enjoying a healthy quality of life throughout our golden years:

DaVINCI DO'S

- Be sure to follow age-related, health-screening guidelines for cancer, heart disease, and other conditions that become more common as we grow older.

- Choose to live a healthy lifestyle by avoiding tobacco, drinking alcohol only in moderation, eating a nutritious diet, exercising daily, getting sufficient sleep (seven to nine hours each night), maintaining an active social life, and engaging your mind to stay sharp and help stave off dementia.

- Consider DNA testing. The technology now exists to screen for about 40 genetic conditions — from aneurysms to cancer. Knowing your own genetic profile can help you adopt healthy lifestyles that can compensate for the specific risks you may face. Diet and exercise have been shown to lower the risk of developing certain cancers, while alcohol can boost cardiovascular health in some people, but may exacerbate health problems in others.

DaVINCI DON'TS

- Don't neglect your dental care. Research shows people with healthy teeth and gums are less likely to develop heart disease and other health problems. Serious oral/dental problems, such gum disease, dramatically increase the risk for cardiovascular problems.

- Never lose track of your health records. If you move to a new state or city, don't forget to ask your doctor, dentist, and other health specialists for records of your health profile, medical data, and any conditions you may have or be predisposed to developing because of genetics or lifestyle. Having those in hand can help you work with your new doctor to customize your healthcare, reduce your risks, and diagnose problems early

- Don't underestimate the connection between stress and health (physical and mental), and be sure to take active steps to manage day-to-day stressors in your life. Meditate, try yoga, listen to music, power off the cellphone or laptop, put down the TV remote, or find some other way to simply spend a few minutes every day actively disengaging from the stresses of modern living, quieting your mind and relaxing your body.

James Taylor famously said: "The secret of life is enjoying the passage of time." Keep in mind that no one lives forever. Life is about the journey, not the destination. Whether you live to a ripe old age or make an early exit, remember to live in the moment and enjoy what you're doing — and the people around you — right here, right now.

It may be a silly cliché, but remember there are only two days we can do nothing about: yesterday and tomorrow. Or, as A. A. Milne once put it:

"Yesterday is history, tomorrow is a mystery, but today is a gift, that's why we call it the *present*."

ObamaCare: What Boomers Need to Know

OBUMMERCARE. ObozoCare. SlowbamaCare. NObamaCare.

Critics of President Barack Obama's Patient Protection and Affordable Care Act had a field day mocking the bumpy rollout of ObamaCare's main provisions in 2013 and 2014, with a host of comically derisive nicknames entering the public lexicon.

But whether you're a foe or a fan of ObamaCare, the future of the US healthcare system is no joking matter. Chances are that you have serious concerns about how the president's landmark healthcare reform law will affect you, your family, your business, and retirement plans — whether you are a senior on Medicare, a Medicaid recipient, uninsured, receiving health benefits from an employer, have a pre-existing conditions, or are otherwise on your own when it comes insurance coverage.

In fact, general healthcare concerns — and related costs of insurance and coverage — topped the list of retirement worries in the United States, according to Bank of America Corp's Merrill

Lynch, whose 2013 survey polled more than 6,300 Americans aged 45 and older.

A whopping 72 percent of retirees surveyed said serious health problems represented their biggest worry, followed by fears of running out of money and being a burden on their family.

The study, co-conducted with research firm Age Wave, also found more affluent Americans — those with more than $250,000 in investable assets — ranked healthcare expenses their biggest worry (52 percent), compared with those that have less than $250,000 (37 percent).

Baby boomers are right to be concerned about rising health costs and the likelihood that they will outpace wages and income in the years ahead. In fact, a 2013 study by Georgetown University and the AARP Public Policy Institute found that trend is already happening for many retirees and those about to enter retirement.

According to the study, retiree income is projected to fall from 80 percent of average career earnings for current retirees to 73 percent for future retirees. This trend is occurring at the same time healthcare costs are rising sharply, at nearly three times the rate of inflation, as noted in Table 13-1.

What's more, the study found that Americans 65 and older now spend about eight percent of their household income on healthcare expenses — a figure projected to more than double in the decade ahead. Those rising healthcare costs are a key reason many aging boomers are delaying retirement — to keep their employer-sponsored health insurance, according to a recent survey by the Employee Benefit Research Institute.

ObamaCare has deepened concerns about healthcare costs, with many credible and nonpartisan health-policy organizations projecting the new law will only accelerate those trends. There is also widespread confusion among many Americans about how

TABLE 13-1: AVERAGE ANNUAL HEALTHCARE COSTS PER PERSON	
Year	Cost
1990	$2,854
2000	$4,878
2010	$8,402

the Affordable Care Act will affect their healthcare and their pocketbooks.

The botched Oct. 1, 2013, opening of the Health Insurance Exchanges — a key aspect of the new law that aims to provide options for the uninsured, the underinsured, and the uninsurable (due to pre-existing health conditions) — seemed to only confuse Americans more, raising a host of new questions:

- How will the exchanges change the game of choosing insurance?

- Are health plans going to cost more or less than in the past?

- How will federal officials enforce the ObamaCare Individual Mandate that all Americans have health insurance or pay a tax?

- Will the employer mandate, requiring all companies with 50 or more workers to provide health benefits, affect healthcare costs and employer-based policies?

- Are changes to Medicare and Medicaid likely to help or hurt recipients in the long run?

- How does ObamaCare pay for new protections for people with chronic health conditions, those unable to afford coverage, new federal subsidies to help middle-income Americans pay for insurance premiums, and new tax credits for small businesses that provide health benefits?

To answer these and other questions, here are ten things baby boomers need to know about the changing healthcare landscape, the Affordable Healthcare Exchanges, the Individual Mandate, and other aspects of ObamaCare.

No. 1: What are the ObamaCare Affordable Healthcare Exchanges?

The Affordable Healthcare Exchanges — a central pillar of ObamaCare — are state-based and federally-run marketplaces that offer a new way to purchase health insurance if you don't get coverage through your employer, Medicare, Medicaid, or the VA. They also allow small businesses to arrange for insurance for their employees through what are called Small Business Health Options Program (SHOP) exchanges.

All 50 states and the District of Columbia offer qualified plans through a health insurance exchange. More than a dozen states, including New York and California, are running their own exchanges. Thirty-six others have elected to have the federal government run their marketplaces, such as Florida and Texas, or are partnering with the federal government to run their exchanges, including Illinois and Michigan.

Big insurers like Humana, United Healthcare, and Blue Cross Blue Shield are offering plans in most states, but a handful of new players and nonprofit organizations have also entered the market in the past year. Plans and costs vary by state, as well as other factors (including your age, health status, and the type of plan you choose).

For information. To find out what your home state is doing and locate your exchange, visit the federal government website, HealthCare.gov.

By phone. US Department of Health and Human Services agents can provide information over the phone and help you review your options and enroll in a plan. You can also fill out a paper application. Call (800) 318-2596.

Small businesses resources. Small business owners who have questions about the SHOP programs can check the HealthCare.gov website for general information or call (800) 706-7893.

Local help: If the website and phone lines are down or busy, visit LocalHelp.Healthcare.gov to search by city, state, or zip code for local help in weighing your options and signing up for a plan. All states have trained and certified assistants to help. Insurance agents and brokers can also be a useful resources to help you make an informed decision.

No. 2: What Are the Penalties for Not Having Insurance?

Americans who do not have insurance through some means will be required to pay a tax penalty to the IRS as of 2014 — $95 per individual (or one percent of your income, whichever is greater) or $285 per family.

That fine rises in 2015 to $325 per individual (or two percent of income), $975 per family. The penalty maxes out at $695 per individual (or 2.5 percent of income) and $2,085 per family in 2016.

No. 3: What Are the Qualifications for a Federal Health Insurance Subsidy?

ObamaCare provides millions of dollars in federal tax subsidies to help cover the insurance premiums of individuals who sign up for plans through the exchanges. Up to 26 million Americans will be eligible for subsidies.

Households with annual incomes of less than 400 percent of the federal poverty level — $45,960 for an individual, $62,040 for a family of two, and $94,200 for a family of four — qualify for a subsidy. You can calculate how much of a subsidy you may receive by visiting an online calculator created by the Kaiser Family Foundation at Kaiser Family Subsidy Calculator: KFF.org/interactive/subsidy-calculator/.

For example:

- A family of four with an annual income of $90,000 (will pay a maximum of 9.5 percent of that amount — $8,930 per year — for a health insurance premium, with a $4,557 federal tax credit subsidy making up the difference (for a bronze-level plan).

- A family of four with a yearly income of about $30,000 will only pay two percent of their income — about $600 per year — for that same plan, with a $12,887 subsidy making up the difference.

- A 60-year-old couple jointly earning $60,000 per year would pay $5,700 in annual premium costs and qualify for a government tax credit of $10,682 (for a silver plan).

In addition, individuals whose incomes fluctuate — those who work on commission or own small businesses where cash flow rises and falls throughout the year — will need to account for any overpayments or underpayments for federally subsidized health insurance when they file their taxes.

SUBSIDY SUBTLETIES

Even small changes in income can result in big differences in subsidies. For instance, a single person earning $33,000 per year qualifies for a mere $6 monthly federal subsidy, compared to a whopping $500 subsidy if that income is just $3,000 less per year.

Americans who qualify for subsidies can choose to apply them directly to their monthly premium to lower their costs (an advanced tax credit), apply a partial subsidy to their premiums, or receive the full subsidy as a credit at tax time.

In addition, low-income residents in about half the states that plan to expand Medicaid under ObamaCare will qualify for free or low-cost healthcare. Individuals earning up to 133 percent of the poverty line, about $30,000 a year for a family of four — who log onto HealthCare.gov will be directed to Medicaid or the Children's Health Insurance Program (CHIP).

No. 4: What Kinds of Plans Are Offered?

By law, insurers must offer four standardized, federally qualified insurance plans — designated bronze, silver, gold, and platinum. Each plan must cover 10 categories of essential benefits, set by the federal government such as emergency service, prescription drug coverage, preventive care, and mental health treatment, but they vary in cost, as follows:

- **Bronze plans** offer the lowest amount of coverage — 60 percent of medical costs on average — but have the lowest premiums.

- **Silver plans:** 70 percent of costs are covered.

- **Gold plans:** 80 percent of costs are covered.

- **Platinum:** 90 percent of costs are covered, but these plans will obviously carry the highest premiums.

No. 5: Will the Plans Cost More Next Year?

The short answer for most baby boomers: Yes.

Some individuals, including older Americans and those with pre-existing conditions, may see a reduction in costs and premiums over time. Americans with pre-existing conditions, who typically paid more for insurance in years past are paying far less as of 2014, because ObamaCare bars insurers from rejecting individuals with medical conditions, such as diabetes, a past cancer diagnosis, high blood pressure, or heart disease. Insurance companies are also barred from charging people with such conditions more for care or setting annual and lifetime caps on coverage.

ObamaCare also bars insurers from raising premiums for policies on individuals after they receive a diagnosis for a chronic condition; this trend was common before the law passed, with many Americans having experienced a rise in premiums after developing cancer, diabetes, or heart disease.

This is a big deal for boomers. According to the Commonwealth Fund, a New York-based private foundation, about 20 percent of Americans in the 50-to-64 age-group went without health insurance for at least part of 2012 — up from 15 percent in 2005 — in part because of pre-existing conditions that made them uninsurable or unable to afford the high costs of premiums.

The law also limits premiums on older Americans to no more than three times the amount charged younger, healthier people, and bars insurers from charging women higher premiums than men.

But these provisions don't mean premiums won't rise overall. In fact, the average costs for healthcare and insurance premiums are projected to increase over the next decade for most Americans, in part because of new consumer protections and standards insurers and healthcare providers must meet as a result of ObamaCare.

According to the latest federal government projections, healthcare costs in the United States are expected to rise 5.8 percent annually between 2014 and 2022. The estimates, by the office of the actuary at the Centers for Medicare and Medicaid Services (part of HHS), project healthcare spending in the United States will grow at a rate that is one percentage point greater than the expected growth in the nation's gross domestic product — a measure of the nation's overall economy. By 2022, healthcare spending will account for nearly one-fifth of the GDP — up from the 2011 level of 17.9 percent, according to the report.

Because ObamaCare contains no cost-control provisions and does not bar insurers from passing on increasing costs to consumers and businesses, insurance premiums and out-of-pocket consumer costs for care are sure to climb in the years ahead, many experts say.

The costs for health plans offered through the new exchanges in the first year of the marketplaces' operation varied widely for individuals and businesses alike, depending on a variety of factors, including age, income, and state of residence. HHS figures show the national average cost for an insurance plan offered through the exchanges for 2014 to be about $328/month. States with the highest insurance costs tend to be those with large rural populations — Wyoming ($516/month), Alaska ($474), and Mississippi ($448). Among the least expensive: Minnesota ($192) and Tennessee ($245).

Some states, such as Florida and Texas, have enormous variations in costs and plans, even within a state's borders. Florida plans, for instance, are right at the national average ($328), but range from $239 to $352 per month, depending on where a resident lives. Texas's monthly rates are slightly below the national average, but a young person living in Austin has seventy-six plans to choose from (averaging $169 per month for lowest-cost option) and one in Dallas-Fort Worth will have forty-three plans (lowest cost option: $217).

In the years ahead, some healthcare analysts say uncertainties may lead to higher price spikes and premium increases down the road, if large numbers of older, sicker people sign up for coverage through the exchanges and small numbers of younger, healthier individuals opt out of such plans.

Federal officials estimate at least seven million younger, healthy Americans, who use fewer healthcare services, will need to buy insurance policies through the exchanges to supplement the health costs for older, sicker individuals (who use more services than their premiums typically cover) for the ObamaCare books to balance.

If not, that could lead to increased insurers' costs that will likely be passed along to policyholders in the form of higher premiums in the years to come.

No. 6: Will Coverage Differ From Past Insurance Policies?

Yes. Choices of doctors, healthcare providers, networks, and drugs are much more limited in some of the newer plans, with insurers seeking to hold down costs by using fewer hospitals and doctors. That's why it's important to check the in-network list of doctors, hospitals, providers, and authorized prescription drugs covered under any plan before you enroll.

You should also calculate key costs, such as premiums, copays, co-insurance, and out-of-pocket limits, before making a selection.

No. 7: What Does the Insurance Application Process Involve?

Online, the application process is automated, but has been complicated by technological and logistical problems in the early going.

HHS has devised a three-page application (down from the original 21 pages) for individuals to apply (online or on paper). You will need to provide the following types of information:

- Name and personal facts (address, Social Security number, date of birth)

- Health status (pregnant, physical/mental conditions)

- Employment status and household income level (using pay stubs or W-2 forms)

- Current health insurance coverage (if any)

- Permission to give an authorized representative, or "navigator," access to application information

No. 8: What About Small Businesses?

Employers with 50 or fewer workers are able to shop for coverage for their employees through the so-called Small Business Health Options Program (SHOP), which is a part of the healthcare exchanges.

The SHOP program aims to level the playing field for small businesses, which have typically paid more than large companies to insure their workers, by pooling them together so they bargain with insurance companies as a single, statewide group. The nonpartisan Congressional Budget Office estimates the SHOP exchanges will lower annual premiums for businesses by one to four percent.

But as with other aspects of ObamaCare, there have been problems with the rollout of the SHOP exchanges.

In late 2013, the Obama administration delayed the full implementation of the SHOP program until 2015, citing logistical problems in getting the small-business exchanges up and running in the first year of operation. Under the delay, small businesses won't be able to use the federal government's health-insurance website — HealthCare.gov — until November 2014 in the 36 states where the federal government is running insurance exchanges or partnering with the states to run them. Businesses can use brokers or enroll directly with insurers in the meantime.

But despite the delay, small businesses with fewer than 25 workers can obtain a tax credit for as much as 50 percent of the cost of insurance for their workforce, as of Jan. 1, 2014 — up from 35 percent in 2013.

In 2016, companies with 100 or fewer employees will be able to arrange insurance through the SHOP exchanges.

No. 9: Is There Any Way Around ObamaCare?

Yes and no. Some individuals are exempt from the Individual Mandate, including Native Americans (covered through the Indian Health Service), prison inmates, millions of individuals with health policies that have been "grandfathered" even though they don't meet ObamaCare's new standards, and a number of business groups, unions, and organizations that have been granted exemptions.

One key exception is for members of so-called "healthcare sharing ministries" — faith-based plans that allow Americans with a common set of ethical or religious beliefs to collect donations from members (such as church parishioners) and share medical bills.

Although such programs are not technically insurance plans, they are allowed under ObamaCare as alternatives. Members decide what procedures will — and won't — be covered. For example, those practices that don't square with an organization's religious or spiritual beliefs, such as contraception or abortion, are usually not covered. Participants also vow to live a Christian lifestyle, swearing off drugs, alcohol, and tobacco.

Members of these co-op plans pay a certain amount of money every month that goes to others in the plan who need help with medical bills. That monthly cost is typically lower than a conventional insurance plan. Medi-Share, the largest Christian health-insurance alternative, has reported that the monthly fees members pay average less than $300 a month for a family plan.

To be exempt from ObamaCare, the plans must have been in existence before the year 2000 and are subject to an independent, publicly available annual audit of their books. Tens of thousands of Americans now belong to Christian health-sharing ministries, but those numbers may grow in the years ahead, experts say.

No. 10: What Are the Smartest Ways to Budget and Plan for Healthcare Costs in Retirement?

Your best defense against rising healthcare costs and premiums as you approach and enter retirement is to come up with a solid offensive strategy — based on what you expect your health and insurance costs are likely to be.

The typical couple with average drug expenses will need about $270,000 to cover medical costs alone throughout retirement, according to a Bankrate.com analysis based on calculations provided by OptumHealth Financial, a United HealthCare Company. Medical costs can be much higher for people who are suffering from certain health conditions, such heart disease, cancer, or diabetes. For example, a person who smokes, has high cholesterol, and is obese may need as much as $150,000 more than a healthy, nonsmoker for healthcare expenses in retirement, according to Bankrate.com.

Of course such costs don't include other healthcare-related expenses, including doctor visits, hospitalizations, and treatments for chronic conditions that may be only partially covered by health plans.

Having health insurance or Medicare can help provide peace of mind. But it's also a good idea to take the following steps to maximize your healthcare dollar:

EXPLORE HEALTH SAVINGS ACCOUNTS

HSAs are tax-free savings accounts that can be used to pay for qualifying out-of-pocket medical expenses not covered by insurance. They can only be used in conjunction with HSA-eligible, high-deductible insurance plans. For 2013, the IRS set the annual limit on deductions at $3,250 for an individual and $6,450 for families. If you're 55 and older, you can contribute an additional $1,000. Unlike a flexible spending account, you don't lose HSA money you don't use in a calendar year; it rolls over year-to-year and can be used to pay for healthcare as well as long-term care. But there are limitations. Under ObamaCare, HSA funds can no longer be used to buy over-the-counter drugs without a doctor's prescription. And those who withdraw HSA funds for nonmedical purposes will see their tax penalty double, from 10 percent to 20 percent of the total withdrawal. But despite the new restrictions on HSAs, they are still a good way to save on your taxes, particularly for people who start contributing to an HSA early and keep adding to their accounts over a period of years.

CONSIDER LONG-TERM CARE INSURANCE

Healthcare and long-term care costs are why nearly one in four Medicare recipients depletes all of his/her savings in the final years of life. Having long-term care insurance can help. It's cheaper to buy long-term care insurance before age 60.

RESOLVE TO STAY HEALTHY

Adopting a healthy lifestyle and taking care to manage any chronic conditions can lower your healthcare costs. Eat a healthy diet, exercise, visit a doctor regularly, and account for any unique personal, familial, or lifestyle factors that can increase your health risks, such as smoking, drinking to excess, being overweight, or not getting adequate sleep.

MANAGE ANY CHRONIC CONDITIONS YOU HAVE

The Centers for Disease Control and Prevention estimates that more than a million Americans have been diagnosed with diabetes, and another five million have it and don't know it. One in nine deaths in the United States is attributed to heart failure, causing more than 279,000 deaths each year, according to the American Heart Association. And rates of cancer are expected to rise to 22.2 million people worldwide by 2030 (from 12.8 million in 2008), according to the American Association for Cancer Research, with one person dying from cancer every minute of every day. But many of the nation's biggest killers, which most often strike after age 55, are preventable. Health experts estimate that more than half of such cases are tied to obesity, smoking, poor diet, lack of exercise, and exposure to ultraviolet radiation from tanning beds or direct sunlight.

BECOME A COMPARISON HEALTH SHOPPER

You wouldn't buy a house, car, or even a new TV without comparing costs of what's on the market, yet many people never think about shopping around for good deals on drugs, healthcare, and medical services. If you're paying out of pocket for medical expenses, resolve to compare prices through online resources like MediBid.com, the HealthcareBluebook.com, and Medicare.gov — all of which provide average and customary costs and prices for various healthcare procedures and products. With such information in hand, you can — and should — try to negotiate fair fees for services with your doctor, hospital, or healthcare provider up front. Other consumer organizations, such as the Patient Advocate Foundation, at PatientAdvocate.org, (800) 532-5273, also offer helpful advice on holding down costs for care and treatment.

ITEMIZE MEDICAL DEDUCTIONS ON YOUR TAXES

Working Americans who file for itemized medical expense deductions are facing new restrictions under ObamaCare provisions, but it may still pay to do so, if you hit certain thresholds. Unreimbursed medical expenses must now add up to at least 10 percent of adjusted gross income — up from 7.5 percent, prior to 2013 — for you to take the deduction and save on federal taxes. But if you have high health costs, it may still make sense to itemize your out-of-pocket expenses, as long as you do the math to be sure it will save you on your taxes. In real dollars, a worker earning $60,000 in gross income needs to have at least $6,000 in out-of-pocket health costs to file for the itemized deduction and save on federal taxes.

SAVE ON DRUG COSTS

If you take brand-name medicines, think about switching to generics, which are usually as effective and less costly. You can also ask your doctor to write prescriptions for over-the-counter drugs (allowing them to be covered by insurance or paid for through tax-free HSA funds). As well, ask your doctor about pill-splitting, which can halve your prescription drug costs. And if you're income is low, ask your pharmacist about drug assistance and discount programs that pharmaceutical companies sponsor. A useful, online clearinghouse for such programs is maintained by the non-profit group NeedyMeds at NeedyMeds.org, (800) 503-6897.

INVESTIGATE INSURANCE REBATES

Under ObamaCare, new rules require insurance companies to spend 80-85 cents of every dollar on actual medical care — not on administration, salaries, overhead, or marketing. Those that don't must provide rebates to consumers. Ask your employer or your insurer if you qualify under the program to see if you have any money coming to you.

LOOK INTO EMPLOYER WELLNESS PROGRAMS

ObamaCare allows employers that provide health benefits to set up wellness reward programs within the insurance coverage they offer to employees. If your employer has established such a program, it could mean that you qualify for lower premiums if you participate and meet the personal wellness standards established by your plan. Check with your employer to see what may apply to you.

OTHER SAVINGS OPTIONS

In addition to looking for ways to hold down health-related costs, it may also pay to explore other financial strategies to compensate by managing other investment and spending plans for a more "holistic" approach to personal financial planning. Look for ways to lower your taxes by sheltering more of your income in retirement savings and HSAs. Create a household budget and stick to it. Clip coupons. Look for two-for-one bargains. Resolve to become a savvy comparison shopper and make an effort to negotiate prices for everything you buy.

Healthcare Spending Skyrocketing

Think your medical bills are high now? You ain't seen nothing yet. Federal government estimates show healthcare costs in the United States are projected to grow at annual rate of 5.8 percent between 2014 and 2022.

And ObamaCare is only partly to blame.

The findings, reported by the Office of the Actuary at the Centers for Medicare and Medicaid Services in the journal *Health Affairs*, project healthcare spending will account for nearly one-fifth of the GDP by 2022.

Based on health spending and economic trends over the past fifty years, future growth in medical expenditures is likely to accelerate as economic conditions improve, the researchers said.

"Although projected growth is faster than in the recent past," said Gigi Cuckler, the lead author of the study, "it is still slower than the growth experienced over the longer term."

By 2022, ObamaCare is projected to reduce the number of uninsured Americans by at least 30 million, increasing overall health spending over the next decade by $621 billion. The increased use of medical services and goods, prescription drugs, and physician and clinical services among the newly insured will boost spending increases in Medicaid (12.2 percent), and private health insurance (7.7 percent), the report said.

Other key findings:

- In 2014, as the major provisions of ObamaCare took effect (including the expansion of Medicaid and the Individual Mandate requiring all Americans to have insurance) growth in spending is expected to hit 6.1 percent.

- Many newly insured Americans will be younger and healthier, and are expected to devote a larger share of their healthcare spending to prescription drugs and physician and clinical services, as opposed to hospital spending.

- Medicaid enrollment is expected to increase by 8.7 million people in 2014, with total Medicaid spending projected to grow to $490 billion, as a result of ObamaCare.

- In 2015, national health spending will remain near 6 percent because eight million more Americans will gain insurance coverage through Medicaid or the exchanges, and the pace of economic recovery is expected to increase in 2014–15, with projected growth in the GDP exceeding five percent for the first time since 2006.

- From 2016 to 2018, healthcare spending is projected to average five percent annually and be influenced by an improving economy and increases in disposable income.

- From 2019 to 2022, Medicare expenditures are projected to grow 7.9 percent per year, compared to 7.3 percent annually from 2016 to 2018, as baby boomers continue to enroll in the program.

- Medicaid spending will grow by 7.9 percent on average in 2015 and 2016, and 6.6 percent from 2017 to 2022, primarily because of an increasing proportion of older and disabled Americans.

- From 2016 to 2022, improved economic conditions are expected to result in an average, private health-insurance-spending growth of 5.8 percent per year.

- By 2022, healthcare, financed by federal, state, and local governments, is projected to account for roughly half of all national health expenditures and reach $2.4 trillion. The federal government will account for more than 63 percent of this total, reflecting expanded Medicaid and Medicare enrollment, and federal subsidies offered through the Affordable Healthcare Exchanges.

Avoiding ObamaCare Scams

ObamaCare has opened the door to scam artists in many regions of the country, as confusion over the new healthcare system, particularly among older Americans, has left many wondering what's required.

In late 2013, California authorities shut down ten bogus ObamaCare websites that mimicked the official "Covered California" affordable health insurance program. Other reports across the country have identified scam artists hawking fake "ObamaCare cards," posing as government employees offering assistance, and creating phony websites that look like the official HealthCare.gov site consumers can use to sign up for insurance plans through the new marketplaces.

Here's what you need to know about three common ObamaCare scams and how to protect yourself.

BOGUS OBAMACARE CARDS

The Better Business Bureau reports many consumers have filed complaints over phone calls they have received by individuals claiming to be government officials offering new health insurance cards they say are required by ObamaCare. Consumers are asked to provide bank account and Social Security numbers to receive their cards. But the truth is, there's no such thing as an ObamaCare card and such pitches are scams. Individuals authorized to provide legitimate ObamaCare assistance can be identified by going through the HHS website, HealthCare.gov, or calling (800) 318-2596.

FRAUDULENT OBAMACARE WEBSITES

Bogus websites, such as the phony Pennsylvania Health Exchange and others of its type in Massachusetts and elsewhere, have been popping up across the country, masquerading as online resources run by insurance companies and regulators, according to the web-based, consumer safety organization, Fraud.org. Also visit the Federal Trade Commission's website for information on ObamaCare scams at Consumer.FTC.gov/articles/0394-suspect-health-care-scam.

MEDICARE SCARE PLOYS

Consumer affairs officials in Florida, California, and other states with large senior populations have reported cases of fraudsters offering to help sign up residents on Medicare for coverage through ObamaCare. AARP has received similar complaints about con artists telling seniors they are about to lose their Medicare coverage or that ObamaCare is replacing their plans. The scammers bank on many seniors falsely believing Medicare benefits are changing under ObamaCare.

To protect yourself from such scams, identity theft experts recommend the following precautions:

- Never give personal information, such as such as credit card numbers, bank account numbers, date of birth, or social security numbers to anyone who contacts you unsolicited by phone, e-mail, social media, or in person.

- Should you receive a solicitation by phone, hang up, don't press any buttons, and don't call back. Likewise, don't reply to any e-mails if you aren't absolutely positive that you know the sender.

- Be aware that government agencies communicate primarily through the mail.

- For legitimate information on the Affordable Care Act, go to HealthCare.gov; for bona fide details on Medicare, visit Medicare.gov.

- Work with reputable insurance agents or legitimate websites (such as esurance.com).

- If you aren't certain whether a website is legit or not, contact your state's Department of Insurance or call officials at the US Department of Health and Human Services at (800) 318-2596.

- If you have mistakenly given information to someone you think is trying to rip you off, contact your bank, credit card providers, and the three major credit bureaus — TransUnion, Experian, and Equifax — to monitor for potential identity thieves. Report any suspected ObamaCare-related scam by calling (800) 318-2596.

14

Quality of Life

ENCOMPASSING EXTERNAL, or physical conditions (health, wealth, environment), and internal, or spiritual conditions (personal contentment, peace of mind, etc.), quality of life is a very subjective concept. We can all imagine the average American tourist visiting a third world country, gazing in wonder and horror at destitute but joyously happy villagers. We can appreciate that standard of living is different from quality of life, but where does true happiness lie? Happiness is closer to self-fulfillment than to mere pleasure, according to Aristotle.

Quality of life was batted around by ancient Greek philosophers before it was more or less taken over by the medical profession. Medical doctors see quality of life or general well-being as something to be evaluated in the context of nutrition, sanitary living conditions, mental ability, and other factors. If you are without illness and healthy, chances are you are also happy.

But "quality of life" is a term used in sociology and economics, as well as by new age gurus of various stripes. Sociologists broadened the scope of the external factors under consideration by studying such elements as access to education, relative standard of living, overall health, and the factors that influence a healthy lifestyle. Quality of life is subjective, but sociologists try to measure the sense of well-being across populations, with Danish work of particular prominence. The Quality of Life Research Center in Copenhagen was established in 1993. In the United States, similarly-named institutions can be found as part of or in association with universities (Carnegie-Mellon, Temple, Claremont, et al.), but also thinly credentialed resorts, spas, and retreats.

One of the underpinnings of quality-of-life studies is the 1962 book by Abraham Maslow, *Towards a Psychology of Being*. Maslow's fundamental idea is that when we take responsibility for our lives, rather than accepting what nature and society seem to have dished out, we use more of our hidden potential and become "self-actualized." Self-actualization is a concept borrowed not only from Aristotle, but from a much older tradition: Buddhism. Today, the interest in quality of life remains dominated by health matters (nutrition and exercise), with a good dollop of spirituality thrown in. In a nutshell, there is no single focus of expertise on quality of life. One deduction that emerges is that fullness and balance pretty much dictates variety.

The vagueness of the term "quality of life" and the relative free-for-all in studying the subject is disturbing to some, including policy-makers who are tasked with allocating public money to research and to actual programs. Here is a summary of one critique of our current concept and measure of quality of life, from the Center of Health Services and Nursing Research, University of Leuven, Belgium:

> Over the past decades, the concept of quality of life has been of paramount importance for evaluating the quality and outcome of healthcare. Despite its importance, there is still no consensus on the definition or proper measurement of quality of life. Several concept analyses of quality of life have been published. However, they appear to have had a rather limited impact on how empirical studies are conducted. Therefore,

we present an overview and critique of different conceptualisations of quality of life, with the ultimate goal of making quality of life a less ambiguous concept.

We also describe six conceptual problems. These problems were used as criteria to evaluate the appropriateness of different conceptualisations. This evaluation suggests that defining quality of life in terms of life satisfaction is most appropriate, because this definition successfully deals with all the conceptual problems discussed. The result of our concept evaluation was not surprising, for it corroborated the results of several concept analyses and the findings of a structural equation modelling study. Based on the findings revealed by our review, we propose that the scientific community should revitalise the conceptual discussion on quality of life. Furthermore, our findings can assist researchers in developing more rigourous quality-of-life research. (NCBI.NLM.NIH .gov/pubmed/16696978.)

What this rather dense excerpt says is that quality of life can best be measured by what people report as "life satisfaction," as determined by research proving that having this criterion met trumps all other categories measured when considering quality of life. Further, the scientific community should accept this new definition going forward. In other words, you can be in dreadful health and living under awful conditions, but if you feel happy, you have a high quality of life.

Economists don't buy it; they prefer measurable indicators like GDP (gross domestic product) per capita, but they also understand that simply being rich doesn't make you happy any more than being happy makes you rich. An interesting twist on economic measurements came from an unlikely corner of the world — the former king of Bhutan, Jigme Singye Wangchuck. The king proposed a measure he named "gross national happiness (GNH)" that would include non-monetary factors like psychological well-being, community vitality, environmental quality, balanced time use over 24 hours, and cultural mores. "If we want our lives to be holistic, our measures of progress should be broader," asserts Karma Ura, the Director of the Center for Bhutan Studies. (NYTimes.com/

roomfordebate/2013/01/16/when-growth-is-not-a-good-goal/
measure-gross-national-happiness.)

The concept of gross national happiness is considered a new economic paradigm that has been discussed at UN conferences, among other places. You can see the criteria used by the center at GrossNationalHappiness.com.

So far GNH has not caught on in a big way, although the Office of National Statistics in the United Kingdom is developing new measures to supplement existing economic and social indicators in order to broaden the picture of society's overall happiness factor. The website of the statistics agency offers data, articles, and video at ONS.gov.uk/ons/guide-method/user-guidance/well-being/index.html.

This pragmatic approach is taken several steps further by *The Economist* magazine, whose Intelligence Unit devised a quality of life index that is much respected and far more useful to the average person, not to mention the average policy-maker. The key goal, for an economist as well as the layman, is to blend the subjective surveys about life-satisfaction with hard facts about material well-being that can be measured in the conventional way, such as income. (Economist.com/media/pdf/QUALITY_OF_LIFE.pdf.)

The core problem is that GDP per capita is "hard" data, but too limited a measure, while sentiment surveys are too squishy and non-verifiable. How do you blend them? GDP per capita is hardly an adequate measure of a broader sense of well-being, since it cannot include nuances like environmental pollution, lack of civil rights, and other immeasurable factors. Besides, who gets to choose what modifying factors we would apply, and how should they be weighted?

The Economist takes the sentiment surveys as a starting point and derives weights for the "hard" factors from the surveys. Applying the weights, the researchers found nine factors that merged well with the satisfaction surveys. In order of importance, they are:

1. Material well-being (GDP per capita)

2. Health (life expectancy at birth)

3. Political stability and security (continuity of government)

4. Family Life (divorce rate)

5. Community life (membership in social organizations)

6. Climate and geography (average temperature and rainfall)

7. Job Security (unemployment rate)

8. Political freedom (political and civil liberties)

9. Gender equality (male to female earnings)

The weightings result in a quality of life index that modifies the satisfaction surveys. Some of the findings are a little surprising at first, but then make perfect sense. For example: "Studies have often found at most a small correlation between education and life-satisfaction, over and above any impact that education has on incomes and health, and possibly other variables such as the extent of political freedom. A recent report by the ILO (International Labor Organization) found that an indicator of schooling and training was actually inversely related to well-being when jobs are poorly attuned to people's needs and aspirations." In other words, a well-paying job will not increase your life satisfaction if you hate it.

Another finding is that money counts. GDP per capita explains about two-thirds of the variation in life-satisfaction across countries, and the relationship is linear. That means that the richer people in one country are, the happier they are than those with lower incomes in the same country. But, getting richer doesn't bring with it a proportionate rise in life-satisfaction in the subjective surveys. Incomes increase faster than satisfaction. In other words, you can be too rich.

The Economist publishes its quality of life index for 130 countries, using a scale of one to 10, with the latest version in November 2012. The magazine says the eleven factors explain 85 percent of the variation in the subjective, life-satisfaction survey scores. While the United States came first in a 1988 version of the index, in 2012, the United States came in 16th, after Switzerland (No. 1), Denmark (No. 5), Canada (No .9) and Ireland (No. 12).

The Economist writes, "Despite their economic dynamism, none of the BRIC countries (Brazil, Russia, India, and China) score impressively. Among the 80 countries covered, Nigeria comes last: it is the worst place for a baby to enter the world in 2013."

"Quibblers will, of course, find more holes in all this than there are in a chunk of Swiss cheese. America was helped to the top spot back in 1988 by the inclusion in the ranking of a 'philistine factor' (for cultural poverty) and a 'yawn index' (the degree to which a country might, despite all its virtues, be irredeemably boring). Switzerland scored terribly on both counts. In the film *The Third Man*, Orson Welles's character, the rogue Harry Lime, famously says that Italy for 30 years had war, terror, and murder under the Borgias but in that time produced Michelangelo, Leonardo da Vinci, and the Renaissance; Switzerland had 500 years of peace and democracy — and produced the cuckoo clock."

So, with centuries of philosophical musing, medical measurements, sociological studies, and adjustments to economic data, it all boils down to one thing: If you feel happy, fulfilled, and satisfied with your life, you are. This is so even if someone else thinks you are living in appalling poverty, ill-health, political oppression, and a lousy climate.

One Size Does Not Fit All

Keep this in mind as you review the advertisements and articles about what you should do and where and how you should live in retirement: One size does not fit all. *The Economist* index offers a clue that the best place to live, if you are planning to relocate abroad, is the one that is the cheapest, even if some of the other conditions (like climate) are not high on your list. But even then, on your own personal checklist, the hot climate may be a more powerful factor than cost of living.

In any case, *The Economist's* index was designed to compare quality of life across countries, not across states, and like all survey averages, may not be representative of your own personal preferences. Declining to move across the country in order to stay close to your family and community may well be the better decision; for most of us these relationships are pretty high on the well-being, factor-list. That doesn't mean you personally should avoid leaving your family and community — just that for most people, having those relationships is a big contributor to a sense of satisfaction in life. As for personal security, it may come quite far down the list, but you probably wouldn't trade

TABLE 14-1: CHEAPEST PLACES TO LIVE (UNDER $40K/YEAR)		
City	**With Mortgage**	**Renter**
Albuquerque, NM	$1150	$657
Augusta, GA	$1064	$626
Columbia, SC	$1107	$712
Jackson, MS	$1053	$624
Knoxville, TN	$1060	$625
Little Rock, AR	$1059	$656
Louisville, KY	$1068	$573
Pittsburgh, PA	$1079	$590
St. Louis, MO	$1186	$657
San Antonio, TX	$1155	$660

Source: http://money.usnews.com/money/retirement/articles/2012/10/15/best-places-to-retire-for-under-40000

it for cheap housing in Detroit, where you can buy a big house for $100, but probably not in a neighborhood where you would feel safe.

Best Places to Live

Obviously there is no single "best" place to live. What is good, better, and best is a function of your preferences and not the preferences of the respondents to a survey. Having said that, you can find an ever-changing list of best places at various websites, including AARP.com and MarketWatch.com.

USNews.com has a list for cheapest places to live for under $400,000 (data is from 2011):

Valuing factors other than cost, AARP.com offers "10 Great Cities for Older Singles," "10 Charming Small Cities you'll Love," and "10 Cool and Quirky Places to Retire."

A final resource is GreatPlacesToRetire.com, which takes 99 towns and cities and compares them for twenty quality-of-life characteristics, including home price, air and water quality, taxes, crime, access to medical care, climate, and cost of living. You can select your own ranking for each of the characteristics to find the town or city best suited to your preferences.

Kiplinger also has "The 10 Most Tax-Friendly States for Retirees." The same site, as well as many others, list the "10 Best Cities for Cheapskates," boasting below-average living costs, an

TABLE 14-2: KIPLINGER TOP TEN CITIES LISTS

10 Cheapest Cities to Live	10 Best Cities for Cheapskates (2012)	10 Best Cities for Cheapskates (8/2013)
1 Idaho Falls, ID	1 St. Louis, MO	1 Omaha, NE
2 Conway, AR	2 El Paso, TX	2 Ogden, UT
3 Springfield, IL	3 Springfield, IL	3 Des Moines, IA
4 Pueblo, CO	4 Kalamazoo, MI	4 Columbus, OH
5 Wichita Falls, TX	5 Spokane, WA	5 Raleigh, NC
6 Fayetteville, AR	6 San Antonio, TX	6 Cincinnati. OH
7 Memphis, TN	7 Eau Claire, WI	7 Sake Lake City, UT
8 Norman OK	8 South Bend, ID	8 Austin, TX
9 McAllen, TX	9 Jonesboro, AR	9 St. Louis, MO
10 Haingten, TX	10 Wichita, KS	10 Cedar Rapids, IA

Source: Kiplinger.com

abundance of public libraries and museums, and a dollar store within a ten-mile radius.

Staying Connected

As discussed briefly in Chapter 4, remaining socially connected — whether with family, friends, significant others, or within social organizations — is paramount to our sense of well-being. As you move into retirement and beyond, many lose spouses, either to death or divorce, children move away, and family members and friends may be busy with their own lives or may have passed on as well. Without a job and seemingly infinite time on your hands, it's easy to isolate ourselves from social situations. Sometimes a disability or medical condition makes it more difficult to partake in social events. Soon enough, you find yourself spending more and more time alone, and that quickly gives way to depression; depressed individuals are prone to lethargy, which leads to atrophy, and ultimately, debilitating health conditions.

If physical activity is exercise for the body, then social activity is exercise for the soul, and we all need a healthy balance of both, among other things, to feel happy and fulfilled. A sense of belonging — being part of something greater than ourselves — is infinitely beneficial to our self-esteem. Getting involved not only lifts our spirits, but keeps our minds agile and can actually add years to our lives. Just like any other age group, there are many ways for early retirees and seniors to become socially involved. In fact, studies show that maintaining a strong social network is a consistent trait of those who live to 100 and beyond.

VOLUNTEER

Giving back to our community provides us with a rewarding sense of fulfillment, and there are countless ways in which you could apply your time and skills to help the less fortunate, such as taking part in literacy programs; community beautification initiatives; tutoring and mentor programs; providing help to troops, veterans, and their families; working in soup kitchens or homeless shelters; or volunteering at hospitals or nursing homes. Research published by the American Psychological Association found that those whose volunteer efforts are solely altruistic may live longer than others whose are not, or those who don't take part at all. Follow these links or call to find an opportunity in which you can do the most good:

- **NationalService.gov/programs/senior-corps/rsvp:** Geared toward those over 55, the federally sponsored Retired and Senior Volunteer Program's (RSVP) website allows you to search for opportunities by interest, state, and zip code. Call **(202) 606-5000, (800) 833-3722 (TTY).**

- **SeniorTransportation.net/ResourcesPublications/Volunteer Transportation:** Utilize private or agency-owned vehicles to provide the elderly and disabled with transportation to doctor's appointments, grocery shopping, social services, etc. Call **(866) 528-6278.**

- **HowStuffWorks.com/economics/volunteer/retired-volunteer-programs:** This article offers boomers top ideas for getting involved, like taking part in disaster relief efforts or legal advocacy.

- **VolunteerMatch.org:** Just as the name implies, Volunteer Match hooks you up with opportunities that best suit your goals and skills. Call **(415) 241-6868.**

Some of these websites, as well as many others tout volunteer travel, or "voluntourism," as a way of aiding the many suffering around the globe, but remember: There is almost always an investment involved. The following CNN.com article showcases free or low-cost voluntourism experiences: CNN.com/2011/09/12/travel/vounteer-free-travel.

GROUPS AND CLUBS

If you can imagine it, chances are it exists. From church groups and playing bridge or chess, to ballroom dancing or bug collecting, folks are getting together as you read, in all corners of the globe, to enjoy shared hobbies and experiences. You can simply go online and search any group, city, and state (e.g., duck hunting enthusiasts, Portland, OR), or try the following to get you on your way:

- **SeniorMeetups.com:** Sign up (for free) using your Facebook or e-mail, and gain access to thousands of opportunities to socialize and/or share activities with like-minded individuals. When you search senior meet-up groups or a similar phrase online, you'll notice that Senior-Meetups.com typically occupies at least the first three hits. An extremely comprehensive nationwide service, they seem to have the meet-up market cornered — virtually a one-stop, meet-up shop. And what's more: You could even start your own meet-up group!

DON'T NEGLECT YOUR PHYSICAL HEALTH

Why not parlay your social activity into an opportunity to get or stay physically fit.

- **SilverSneakers.com:** The nation's leading exercise program for active adults offers free memberships to qualifying seniors at over 11,000 fitness centers across the country. To quote their website, "If you're a group retiree or part of a Medicare health plan, you may already have a Silver Sneakers membership." Memberships also include classes, such as yoga, and outdoor exercise activities like nature walks. Even if you're not a group retiree or Medicare recipient, you may still qualify. Call (888) 423-4632, (TTY: 711).

If going to a gym isn't quite your style, considering joining a senior sports or recreational league. Playing on a team or as part of a league offers great possibilities for meeting new people — and having fun doing something that's good for you at the same time. Check out USTA.com, (800) 990-8782, to connect with local tennis players. Visit the National Golf Foundation website, NGF .org, or call (561) 744-6006 for resources, clubs, and connections. Can't decide on a particular sport? Join YMCA or a health spa that offers anything from yoga, aqua aerobics, or other activities to help you decide what interests you. For more information, visit the International Health, Racquet & Sportsclub Association website at IHRSA.org, or call (800) 228-4772.

DATING OVER 50

Don't give up on romance. If you've recently (or not so recently) divorced, or are a widow or widower, there's no reason to believe that you're doomed to live out the rest of your days alone. Such life changes can be devastating, but once we've gone through the healthy and necessary range of emotions on the road toward healing, we may begin to once again yearn to have someone by our side. As we mature, we get to know ourselves better, as well as having a better handle on what we'd like in a partner. So your second (third, or even fourth) time around might be even better than the first. The following are some sites that may help you make a love connection, or at the very least, meet a new friend.

- Match.com

- OurTime.com

- SeniorMatch.com

- SeniorFriendFinder.com

- BoomerMatchup.com

ADOPT A PET

For those of us who'd prefer to fly solo, a pet is a great solution to ward off loneliness. For years we've been hearing about studies surrounding the many health benefits of owning a pet, especially where single retirees and seniors are concerned. Pets are proven to reduce stress levels, which in turn lowers blood pressure. As well, Fido or Mittens can provide us with companionship, and the responsibility of caregiving diverts attention away from ourselves, allowing us to put our problems and ailments aside. For those of us who live alone, adopting a pet is a proven way to combat depression. Call the American Humane Association at (800) 227-4645, or go online to find a shelter in your area: AmericanHumane.org.

Time Well-Spent

Something big that is missing from *The Economist's* and *Forbes'* lists is what we generally call "hobbies." This is a semantically loaded word that can imply an amateurish activity that is little more than a distraction and produces nothing of real value. To say that a retired person has a hobby skates close to being insulting, when in practice, some hobbyists are the leading figures in their fields. It was a retired Japanese man who advanced robotics, and many a retired person has contributed to open-source software. Every single one of those articles on "Eight Steps to a Successful Retirement" and "The 5 Top Habits of Happy Retirees" contains an item that pertains to staying actively involved in some activity that interests you, even if it's not a money-making hobby.

Maybe beer-making at home is not for you, and neither are wood-carving, stamp-collecting, or growing organic vegetables for the farmers' market. With any luck, you like to read:

> The best thing . . . is to learn something. That's the only thing that never fails. You may grow old and trembling in your anatomies, you may lie awake at night listening to the disorder of your veins, you may miss your only love, you may see the world about you devastated by evil lunatics, or know your honor trampled in the sewers of baser minds. There is only one thing for it then — to learn. Learn why the world wags and what wags it. That is the only thing which the mind can never exhaust, never alienate, never be tortured by, never fear or distrust, and never dream of regretting. Learning is the only thing for you. Look what a lot of things there are to learn.
>
> Merlin, in T. H. White's, *The Once and Future King*

Living Long *and* Healthy

When Nelson Mandela died in December 2013, his passing drew a global outpouring of emotion, tributes, and celebrations that honored his noble life's work as a human rights activist, political visionary, community leader, and peaceful freedom fighter.

But in a sidelight to the international coverage of Mandela's passing, health experts pointed to another important legacy of the South African leader's life that should be a lesson to us all: The community activism for which he will be admired and remembered for years to come may also have contributed to his longevity.

There is ample scientific evidence that the kind of positive outlook Mandela maintained — as well as the global connections he made as part of his community activism — may have helped buffer him from the physical stresses and extreme adversity he suffered throughout his life, helping him live to the ripe old age of 95.

Mandela, who helped end apartheid, served as the country's president between 1991 and 1997, after spending twenty-seven hard years in prison. During his incarceration he reportedly experienced malnutrition, including a deficiency of vitamin D, which has been linked to heart disease, diabetes, and other life-threatening health conditions. He was also required to perform hard labor, which can take a significant physical and mental toll.

Yet despite these hardships, he managed to maintain a relentlessly upbeat attitude, connected with people wherever he traveled, and lived to see his 95th birthday (something only about one in every 4,000 Americans achieves, according to US Census data).

Lessons from Centenarians

Many scientific studies of individuals who have lived a century or more have identified predictable health factors that appear to contribute to a longer life. A 2010 study of people 100 years or older found, for instance, that certain genetic markers can predict with a high degree of accuracy whether someone will hit that birthday benchmark. Another study of people living in Sicily found those who lived past the age of 100 closely followed a Mediterranean diet, loaded with fruits, vegetables, and whole grains, and low in red meat and refined carbohydrates.

But scientists are also just beginning to understand the connection between longevity and social and psychological factors — including a positive outlook and close connections with family and friends.

A dozen major studies have been conducted worldwide on centenarians. Most have confirmed the health benefits of exercise, a healthy diet, and staying mentally active. But they have also found building and maintaining close social and family networks to be a consistent trait of most people who live to 100 and beyond.

One possible reason: Close relationships may offer some protection against depression and isolation, which can lead to heart disease, Alzheimer's, and other chronic life-threatening conditions.

Those relationships don't necessarily need to involve close family and friends. A 2013 study by Purdue University found, for instance, that people over 70 years of age who engage in volunteer efforts tend to live longer lives. In addition to the psychological benefits that come from helping other people, the researchers said older adults who regularly volunteer are in better physical health than those just a few years younger — even when other factors (such as diet and exercise levels) are taken into account.

"We looked at older adults engaging in a variety of productive activities, but there is something really distinctive about volunteering that positively affects a person's physical health," said Seoyoun Kim, a doctoral student in sociology and gerontology who led the 2013 study, published in *The Gerontologist*.

To reach their conclusions, Kim's team measured physical health and activities such as volunteering, caregiving, community engagement, and employment of 1,790 independent-living individuals, aged 57–85 years. The researchers also tracked a specific biomarker tied to inflammation in the body that can accurately reflect people's overall health. The C-reactive protein (CRP) increases with age, and higher amounts are associated with many health problems such as cardiovascular disease, diabetes, and some cancers.

The study, known as the *National Social Life, Health and Aging Project*, found that CRP was about 15 percent lower in those who volunteered several times per year than for those who did not.

"We believe we are the first to document this link by measuring chronic inflammation," said Kenneth F. Ferraro, a Purdue professor of sociology. "By using a biomarker, which is like a canary in the mine, we can clinically detect a person's physiological health, whether it has been diagnosed or not."

How might social networks, health, and longevity be related? Kim noted older adults who volunteer remain connected to the communities and continue to build relationships after retiring or raising children.

"Volunteering allows them to engage in meaningful roles and stay active," Kim said. "In gerontology we are interested in people living well as they live longer. The relationship between volunteering and inflammation is telling because it's related to their quality of life and disease prevention."

Ferraro added that community involvement may confer other psycho-social benefits that can boost lifespan and offer protection against life-threatening conditions: "Volunteering helps many people see what is important in life and how fortunate we are. Having the feeling that you are making a difference in a person's life is powerful, and our own problems may not seem so important. I also think volunteering is special because one gets to select the nature of the charitable endeavor. You are not coerced; you have some choice in it."

Ferraro's observations may explain the findings of another study by Johns Hopkins University that determined that people who care for a chronically ill or disabled family member tend to live longer than those who don't — a finding that contradicts long-standing beliefs about the negative health effects of stress on caregivers.

The 2013 study, published in the *American Journal of Epidemiology*, tracked more than 3,500 family caregivers for six years and found they experienced an 18 percent survival advantage, compared to a similar group of individuals who did not care for ill or disabled loved ones.

"Taking care of a chronically ill person in your family is often associated with stress, and caregiving has been previously linked to increased mortality rates," said David L. Roth, director of the Johns Hopkins University Center on Aging and Health. "Our study provides important new information on the issue of whether informal family caregiving responsibilities are associated with higher or lower mortality rates as suggested by multiple conflicting previous studies."

Roth and his colleagues said the study, sponsored by the National Institutes of Health, suggests caregiving, while stressful, may confer some psychological benefits that boost overall health and longevity.

"In many cases, caregivers report receiving benefits of enhanced self-esteem, recognition, and gratitude from their care recipients," said Roth. "Thus, when caregiving is done willingly, at manageable levels, and with individuals who are capable of expressing gratitude, it is reasonable to expect that health benefits might accrue in those situations."

Strive for Balance

Throughout this book, we've covered all of the technicalities integral to creating a sound retirement plan — from calculating life expectancy to savings and the cost of retirement, as well as Social Security, Medicare, wills and trusts, investing, long-term care, advance directives, and beyond. We've examined what is required in planning and budgeting for healthcare — both the expected and unexpected — as well as advice for keeping our bodies nourished and fit. But none of us exists in a vacuum and neither should our retirement plan, and for each of these practical considerations, there exists a facet of equal or greater importance: the human factor.

It is scientifically proven that an orphaned infant, even with its physical needs met and provided with proper nutrition, will die if deprived of human touch and interaction. Likewise, no matter how airtight our retirement strategy with respect to finances and legalities, without a plan in place for nourishing the soul — remaining socially connected, caring for others and being cared for, engaging in activities that feed our spirit and increase self-esteem — our long-anticipated retirement will not only be lonely and lacking in pleasure and quality, but likely unhealthy and brief.

Perfection is an ever-elusive pursuit. Therefore, in lieu of striving for the perfect retirement plan (or perfection in any capacity, for that matter), we urge you, when or if all else fails, to focus on balance — balance in all things. Just as you'd heed the advice of financial advisors when they stress diversity in your investment portfolio, nutritionists when they suggest variety when it comes to your diet, and fitness experts when they say the same regarding your exercise routine, we often neglect other needs that are just as crucial to an overall sense of well-being, health, inner harmony, and wholeness. Those needs and experiences — emotional, spiritual, and intellectual — are what add color, texture, richness, and beauty to our shared life journey. Perhaps Steve Jobs best expressed the value of inner contentedness and fulfillment above all else: "Being the richest man in the cemetery doesn't matter to me. Going to bed at night saying we've done something wonderful, that's what matters to me."

Afterword

THE BABY BOOM GENERATION, perhaps more than any other, redefined American life and lifestyles in ways that forever changed the fabric of the nation's political, social, and cultural climate over the past six decades.

As the generation of Americans born between 1946 and 1964 came of age, the world transformed right along with them — in ways both subtle and dramatic. The cultural and political revolutions of the 1960s were largely driven by young civil-rights-minded boomers questioning authority and all that had gone before. A redefinition of family and family values emerged in the 1970s as boomers became parents and created households that were markedly different from their own childhood experiences. In the 1980s, the generation's embrace of untraditional careers in midlife revolutionized the workplace and conventional employment patterns. And since the 1990s, boomers' embrace of digital media, technology, healthy lifestyles, leisure, and entertainment have continued to ripple through every facet of our society — driving unprecedented change every step of the way.

And so, as boomers enter their golden years, the question is: Why shouldn't it be expected that traditional notions of retirement will also be upended by the generation that has redefined every other aspect and passage of American life?

The answer, of course, is that transformation is already well underway — so much so, in fact, that we may need to come up with a new term for retirement in the boomer era. For many of the 10,000 boomers turning 65 every day in this country, *retirement* actually means something more akin to reinvention or reawakening.

With that in mind, it is our sincere hope that this book has provided the guidance to help you move forward with your own personal reinvention and reawakening in your golden years. We have provided advice and suggestions not just for living, but for living well — financially, socially, physically, and mentally. Now, it's up to you.

As Gail Sheehy, author of the best-selling *Passages*, observes: "If every day is an awakening, you will never grow old. You will just keep growing."

We wish you luck, as your journey continues.

Appendix A:
Unbiased Resources

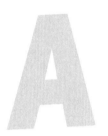

THE INS AND OUTS of Medicare and health-related insurance issues are complicated. But help is available, with a number of nonprofit agencies, patient-advocacy groups, and assistance organizations providing nonbiased information in all 50 states and the District of Columbia.

A good place to start is the State Health Insurance Assistance Program (SHIP), a national initiative that offers free, one-on-one counseling and assistance. ShipTalk.org can help you identify the SHIP program contact information in your state.

All states offer SHIP programs, but they are known by other names in some places. They are funded on both the state-level and by the United States Centers for Medicaid and Medicare Services (CMS) to provide free, objective health-insurance information and one-on-one counseling. What follows is a state-by-state list of SHIP programs and other organizations that offer help to people with Medicare, residents eligible for Medicare, and those seeking information on insurance-related matters (updated through October 2013). ShipTalk.org can also help you identify the SHIP program contact information in your state.

ALABAMA

State Health Insurance Assistance Program
www.adss.alabama.gov/ship.cfm
(800) 243-5463

ALASKA

State Health Insurance Assistance Programs & Senior
Medicare Patrol:
www.dhss.alaska.gov/dsds/Pages/medicare/default.aspx
(800) 478-6065

ARIZONA

State Health Insurance Assistance Program:
www.azdes.gov/daas/ship
(800) 432-4040

ARKANSAS

Senior Health Insurance Information Program:
www.insurance.arkansas.gov/Seniors/divpage.htm
(800) 224-6330, (501) 371-2782

CALIFORNIA

California Department of Aging's Health Insurance
Counseling and Advocacy Program:
www.aging.ca.gov/hicap/default.aspx
(800) 434-0222

COLORADO

Senior Health Insurance Assistance Program:
www.dora.colorado.gov/insurance
(888) 696-7213

CONNECTICUT

Connecticut Health Insurance Assistance, Outreach, Information, Referral, Counseling and Eligibility Screening: www.ct.gov/agingservices/cwp/view.asp?a=2513&q=313032
(800) 994-9422

DELAWARE

ELDERinfo:
www.delawareinsurance.gov/services/elderinfo.shtml
(800) 336-9500, (302) 674-7364

FLORIDA

SHINE (Serving Health Insurance Needs of Elders):
www.floridashine.org
(800) 963-5337

GEORGIA

GeorgiaCares:
www.mygeorgiacares.org
(800) 669-8387

HAWAII

Sage PLUS Program:
www.hawaiiship.org
(808) 586-7299

IDAHO

SHIBA (Senior Health Insurance Benefits Advisors):
www.doi.idaho.gov/shiba/shwelcome.aspx
(800) 247-4422

ILLINOIS

Senior Health Insurance Program:
www.insurance.illinois.gov
(800) 548-9034

INDIANA

Senior Health Insurance Program:
https://www.in.gov/idoi/2500.htm
(800) 452-4800

IOWA

Senior Health Insurance Information Program:
https://www.shiip.state.ia.us/FindACounselor.aspx
(800) 351-4664

KANSAS

Senior Health Insurance Counseling For Kansas:
www.kdads.ks.gov/shick/shick_index.html
(800) 860-5260

KENTUCKY

Kentucky State Health Insurance Information Program:
www.chfs.ky.gov/dail/ship.htm
(877) 293-7447

LOUISIANA

Senior Health Insurance Information Program:
www.ldi.louisiana.gov/Health/SHIIP/index.html
(800) 454-9573

MAINE

Senior Health Insurance Information Program:
www.maine.gov/dhhs/oes/resource/health_insurance.htm
(877) 353-3771

MARYLAND

Senior Health Insurance Information Program:
www.aging.maryland.gov/SeniorHealthInsurance
Program.html
(800) 243-3425, ext. 71108

MASSACHUSETTS

SHINE Program (Serving Health Information Needs of Elders):
www.massresources.org/health-care.html
(800) 243-4636, press 3

MICHIGAN

Medicare/Medicaid Assistance Program:
www.mmapinc.org
(800) 803-7174

MINNESOTA

Minnesota Senior Health Insurance Information Program:
www.health.state.mn.us/ship
(800) 333-2433

MISSISSIPPI

Senior Health Insurance Information Program:
www.mdhs.state.ms.us/aas_ship.html
(800) 948-3090

MISSOURI

Community Leaders Assisting the Insured of Missouri:
www.missouriclaim.org
(800) 390-3330

MONTANA

Montana Senior Health Insurance Information Program:
www.dphhs.mt.gov/sltc/services/aging/SHIP/ship.shtml
(800) 551-3191

NEBRASKA

Nebraska Senior Health Insurance Information Program:
www.doi.nebraska.gov/shiip/
(800) 234-7119

NEVADA

Senior Health Insurance Information Program:
www.nvaging.net/ship/ship_main.htm
(800) 307-4444, Las Vegas: **(702) 486-3478**

NEW HAMPSHIRE

ServiceLink Resource Centers:
www.nh.gov/servicelink/medicareinfo.html
(866) 634-9412

NEW JERSEY

State Health Insurance Information Program:
www.state.nj.us/humanservices/doas/services/ship/
(800) 792-8820

NEW MEXICO

State Health Insurance Information Program:
www.nmaging.state.nm.us/State_Health_Insurance_
Assistance_Program.aspx
(800) 432-2080

NEW YORK

Health Insurance Information, Counseling and Assistance:
www.aging.ny.gov/HealthBenefits/Index.cfm
(800) 701-0501

NORTH CAROLINA

Seniors' Health Insurance Information Program:
www.ncdoi.com/SHIIP/Default.aspx
(800) 443-9354

NORTH DAKOTA

Senior Health Insurance Counseling Program:
www.nd.gov/ndins/shic
(800) 575-6611

OHIO

Ohio Senior Health Insurance Information Program:
www.insurance.ohio.gov/aboutodi/odidiv/pages/oshiip.aspx
(800) 686-1578

OKLAHOMA

Senior Health Insurance Information Program:
www.ok.gov/oid/Consumers/Information_for_
Seniors/SHIP.html
(800) 763-2828

OREGON

Senior Health Insurance Information Program:
www.oregon.gov/DCBS/SHIBA
(800) 722-4134

PENNSYLVANIA

Apprise Health Insurance Counseling Program:
www.portal.state.pa.us/portal/servept?open=
514&objID=616587&mode=2
(800) 783-7067

RHODE ISLAND

Rhode Island Senior Health Insurance Information Program:
www.dea.ri.gov/insurance/
(401) 462-4000

SOUTH CAROLINA

Insurance Counseling Assistance and Referrals for Elders
program (I-CARE):
www.aging.sc.gov/seniors/medicare/Pages/default.aspx
(803) 771-0131

SOUTH DAKOTA

Senior Health Information & Insurance Education (SHIINE):
www.shiine.net
Eastern South Dakota: (800) 536-8197 or (605) 333-3314;
Central South Dakota: (877) 331-4834 or (605) 224-3212;
Western South Dakota: (877) 286-9072 or (605) 342-8635

TENNESSEE

Tennessee State Health Insurance Assistance Program:
www.tn.gov/comaging/ship.html
(877) 801-0044

TEXAS

Health Information Counseling & Advocacy Program of Texas: www.tdi.texas.gov/consumer/hicap/hicaphme.html
(800) 252-3439

UTAH

Medicare/Medigap/Med Advantage: www.daas.utah.gov/senior-services
(801) 538-3800

VERMONT

Vermont State Health Insurance Assistance Program: www.medicarehelpvt.net
(800) 642-5119

VIRGINIA

Virginia Insurance Counseling and Assistance Program: www.vda.virginia.gov/vicap.asp
(800) 552-3402

WASHINGTON

Statewide Health Insurance Benefits Advisors: www.insurance.wa.gov/about-oic/what-we-do/advocate-for-consumers/shiba/
(800) 562-6900

WASHINGTON D.C.

Health Insurance Counseling Project: www.law.gwu.edu/Academics/EL/clinics/insurance/Pages/About.aspx
(202) 739-0668

WEST VIRGINIA

West Virginia State Health Insurance Assistance Program: www.wvship.org/AboutWVSHIP/tabid/132/Default.aspx
(877) 987-4463

WISCONSIN

Medigap Helpline:

www.dhs.wisconsin.gov/aging/EBS/ship.htm

(800) 242-1060

WYOMING

Wyoming State Health Insurance Information Program:

www.wyomingseniors.com/services/

wyoming-state-health-insurance-information-program

(800) 856-4398

Patient Advocates, Insurance Ombudsmen by State

For health insurance issues outside of Medicare and Medicaid, all states have designated ombudsmen or other patient-advocacy divisions that provide assistance and information, and even serve as a forum for resolving medical disputes and problems. Some are more active and offer more resources than others, but they can be a good place to start, if you're looking for general information on insurance or to resolve a complicated dispute.

What follows is a state-by-state listing of insurance divisions, consumer advocacy agencies, and ombudsmen.

ALABAMA

Alabama Department of Insurance

P.O. Box 303351

Montgomery, AL 36130-3351

www.alabamaadministrativecode.state.al.us/

docs/ins/index.html

(334) 269-3550

ALASKA

Alaska Division of Insurance

550 West 7th Avenue, Suite 1560

Anchorage, AK 99501-3567

www.commerce.alaska.gov/dnn/ins/Home.aspx

(907) 269-7900

ARIZONA

Arizona Department of Insurance
2910 North 44th Street, Suite 210
Phoenix, AZ 85018-7269

www.azinsurance.gov
(602) 364-3100

ARKANSAS

Arkansas Insurance Department
Consumer Services Division
1200 West Third Street
Little Rock, AR 72201-1904

www.insurance.arkansas.gov
(501) 371-2600

CALIFORNIA

California Department of Insurance
Office of the Ombudsman
300 Capitol Mall, Suite 1700
Sacramento, CA 95814-0064

www.insurance.ca.gov
(916) 492-3500

COLORADO

Colorado Division of Insurance
1560 Broadway, Suite 850
Denver, CO 80202-4910

www.cdn.colorado.gov/cs/Satellite/DORA-DI/CBON/
DORA/1251623445671
(303) 894-7499

CONNECTICUT

Connecticut Insurance Department
P.O. Box 816
Hartford, CT 06142-0816

https://cidonline.ct.gov/ccf/
(860) 297-3800

DELAWARE

Delaware Department of Insurance
841 Silver Lake Boulevard
Dover, DE 19904-2465

www.delawareinsurance.gov
(302) 674-7300

DISTRICT OF COLUMBIA

District of Columbia Department of Insurance,
Securities, and Banking
Office of Health Care Ombudsman and Bill of Rights
825 North Capitol Street, NE, 6th Floor
Washington, D.C. 20002-2410

www.ombudsman.dc.gov/ombudsman/site/default.asp
?ombudsmanNav_GID=0&ombudsmanNav_GID=1463
(202) 478-1397

FLORIDA

Florida Department of Insurance
Office of Insurance Regulation
The Larson Building
200 E. Gaines Street, Room 101A
Tallahassee, FL 32399-0305

www.apps.fldfs.com/ESERVICE/Default.aspx
(850) 413-5914

GEORGIA

Georgia Department of Insurance
Office of Insurance and Safety Fire Commissioner
2 Martin Luther King, Jr. Drive, West Tower, Suite 704
Atlanta, Georgia 30334-9061

www.oci.ga.gov/ConsumerService/complaintprocess.aspx
(404) 656-2070

HAWAII

Hawaii Department of Insurance
Department of Commerce and Consumer Affairs
Insurance Division
P.O. Box 3614
Honolulu, HI 96811-3614

www.cca.hawaii.gov/ins/
(808) 586-2790

IDAHO

Idaho Department of Insurance
P.O. Box 83720
Boise, ID 83720-0043

www.doi.idaho.gov
(208) 334-4250

ILLINOIS

Illinois Department of Insurance
320 W Washington Street
Springfield, IL 62767-0001

www.insurance.illinois.gov
(217) 782-4515

INDIANA

Indiana Department of Insurance
311 W Washington Street, Suite 300
Indianapolis, IN 46204-2787

www.in.gov/idoi/2552.htm
(317) 232-2385

IOWA

Iowa Department of Insurance
Iowa Insurance Division
330 Maple Street
Des Moines, IA 50319-0065

www.insuranceca.iowa.gov
(515) 281-5705

KANSAS

Kansas Department of Insurance
Kansas Insurance Department
420 SW 9th Street
Topeka, KS 66612-1678

www.ksinsurance.org/
(785) 296-3071

KENTUCKY

Kentucky Department of Insurance
P.O. Box 517
Frankfort, KY 40602-0517

www.insurance.ky.gov
(502) 564-3630

LOUISIANA

Louisiana Department of Insurance
P.O. Box 94214
Baton Rouge, LA 70804-9214

www.ldi.state.la.us/index.html
(225) 342-5900

MAINE

Maine Department of Insurance
Department of Professional & Financial Regulation
Maine Bureau of Insurance
34 State House Station
Augusta, ME 04333-0034

www.maine.gov/pfr/insurance/index.shtml
(207) 624-8475

MARYLAND

Maryland Insurance Administration
200 St. Paul Place, Suite 2700
Baltimore, MD 21202-2093

www.mdinsurance.state.md.us/sa/jsp/Mia.jsp
(410) 468-2090

MASSACHUSETTS

Massachusetts Division of Insurance
Office of Consumer Affairs and Business Regulation
1000 Washington Street, 8th Floor
Boston, MA 02118-6200

www.mass.gov/ocabr/government/oca-agencies/doi-lp/
(617) 521-7794

MICHIGAN

Michigan Department of Insurance & Financial Services
P.O. Box 30220
Lansing, MI 48909-7720

www.michigan.gov/difs
(517) 373-0220

MINNESOTA

Minnesota Department of Insurance
85 7th Place East, Suite 500
St. Paul, MN 55101-2198

www.mn.gov/commerce/insurance/
(651) 296-6025

MISSISSIPPI

Mississippi Insurance Department
P.O. Box 79
Jackson, MS 39205-0079

www.mid.ms.gov
(601) 359-3569

MISSOURI

Missouri Department of Insurance
Financial Institutions and Professional Registration (DIFP)
P.O .Box 690
Jefferson City, MO 65102-0690

www.insurance.mo.gov
(573) 751-4126

MONTANA

Montana Office of the Commissioner of Securities
and Insurance
Montana State Auditor
840 Helena Avenue
Helena, MT 59601-3423

www.csi.mt.gov
(406) 444-2040

NEBRASKA

Nebraska Department of Insurance
P.O. Box 82089
Lincoln, NE 68501-2089

www.doi.nebraska.gov
(402) 471-2201

NEVADA

Nevada Dept. of Business & Industry Division of Insurance
1818 East College Pkwy, Suite 103
Carson City, NV 89706-7986

www.doi.nv.gov
(775) 687-0700

NEW HAMPSHIRE

New Hampshire Insurance Department
21 South Fruit Street, Suite 14
Concord, NH 03301-2428

www.nh.gov/insurance
(603) 271-2261

NEW JERSEY

State of New Jersey Department of Banking and Insurance
20 West State Street
P.O. Box 325
Trenton, NJ 08625-0325

www.state.nj.us/dobi/index.html
(609) 292-7272

NEW MEXICO

New Mexico Public Regulation Commission Division of Insurance
P.O. Box 1689
Santa Fe, NM 87504-1689

www.nmprc.state.nm.us
(505) 827-4601

NEW YORK

New York State Department of Financial Services
One State Street
New York, NY 10004-1511

www.dfs.ny.gov
(212) 709-3500

NORTH CAROLINA

North Carolina Department of Insurance
1201 Mail Service Center
Raleigh, NC 27699-1201

www.ncdoi.com
(919) 733-3058

NORTH DAKOTA

North Dakota Insurance Department
State Capitol, Fifth Floor
600 E. Boulevard Avenue
Bismarck, ND 58505-0320

www.nd.gov/ndins/
(701) 328-2440

OHIO

Ohio Department of Insurance
50 West Town Street Third Floor, Suite 300
Columbus, OH 43215-1067

www.insurance.ohio.gov/Pages/default.aspx
(614) 644-2658

OKLAHOMA

Oklahoma Insurance Department
7645 E. 63rd Street, Suite 102
Tulsa, OK 74133-1249

www.ok.gov/oid/
(918) 295-3700

OREGON

Oregon Department of Consumer & Business Services
Insurance Division
P.O. Box 14480
Salem, OR 97309-0405

www.insurance.oregon.gov
(503) 947-7980

PENNSYLVANIA

Pennsylvania Insurance Department
1326 Strawberry Square
Harrisburg, PA 17120-0046

www.insurance.pa.gov/portal/server.pt/community/
insurance_pa_gov/4679
(717) 783-0442

RHODE ISLAND

Rhode Island Department of Business Regulation
Division of Insurance
1511 Pontiac Avenue, Building 69-2
Cranston, RI 02920-4407

www.dbr.state.ri.us/divisions/insurance/
(401) 462-9520

SOUTH CAROLINA

South Carolina Department of Insurance
P.O. Box 100105
Columbia, SC 29202-3105

www.doi.sc.gov
(803) 737-6160

SOUTH DAKOTA

South Dakota Department of Labor & Regulation Division
of Insurance
445 East Capitol Avenue
Pierre, SD 57501-3185

www.dlr.sd.gov/insurance/
(605) 773-3563

TENNESSEE

Tennessee Department of Commerce & Insurance
Davy Crockett Tower Twelfth Floor
500 James Robertson Parkway
Nashville, TN 37243-0565

www.tn.gov/commerce/
(615) 741-2176

TEXAS

Texas Department of Insurance
P.O. Box 149104
Austin, TX 78714-9104

www.tdi.texas.gov
(512) 463-6169

UTAH

Utah Insurance Department
3110 State Office Building
Salt Lake City, UT 84114-1207

www.insurance.utah.gov
(801) 538-3800

VERMONT

Vermont Department of Financial Regulation
Insurance Division
89 Main Street
Montpelier, VT 05620-3168

www.dfr.vermont.gov/insurance/insurance-division
(802) 828-3301

VIRGINIA

Virginia State Corporation Commission Bureau of Insurance
P.O. Box 1157
Richmond, VA 23218-1157

www.scc.virginia.gov/boi/
(804) 371-9741

WASHINGTON

Washington State Office of the Insurance Commissioner
P.O. Box 40256
Olympia, WA 98504-0256

www.insurance.wa.gov
(360) 725-7000

WEST VIRGINIA

West Virginia Offices of the Insurance Commissioner
P.O. Box 50540
Charleston, WV 25305-0540

www.wvinsurance.gov/#14632-glossary
(304) 558-3354

WISCONSIN

State of Wisconsin Office of the Commissioner of Insurance
P.O. Box 7873
Madison, WI 53707-7873

www.oci.wi.gov
(608) 266-3585

WYOMING

Wyoming Insurance Department
106 East Sixth Avenue
Cheyenne, WY 82002-1312

www.doi.wyo.gov
(307) 777-7401

Appendix B: Assisted-Living Facilities and Nursing Homes

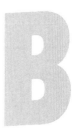

How to Choose an Assisted-Living Facility

Assisted-living facilities are home to nearly one million Americans. Each state has its own licensing regulations and inspections requirements, with little federal oversight of the more than 39,500 facilities in the US. As a result, it's important to thoroughly investigate any facility you are considering for an aging parent or relative. Here are a few tips on choosing an assisted-living facility to get you started:

COMPARE ASSISTED LIVING TO HOME CARE

An assisted-living facility isn't the best option for everyone. Home care might be a better choice for a relative who is still able to manage his or her own affairs, with just a little assistance. Assisted-living facilities are residential units that typically include a kitchen, but staff provides meals, housekeeping, transportation, and other kinds of personal assistance. Costs typically start at about $5,000 a month. For help and information:

- A family physician or geriatric-care specialist can assess a relative's need for comprehensive assisted-living care. Check the website of National Association of Professional Geriatric Care Managers, CareManager.org, (520) 881-8008, for a local specialist.

- The Consumer Consortium on Assisted Living, a nonprofit advocacy group, provides useful information on its website, CCAL.org, (732) 212-9036.

- The National Long-Term Care Ombudsman Resource Center at LTCOmbudsman.org, (202) 332-2275, can provide information about your state's long-term-care ombudsman or resident advocate — as well as a record of complaints lodged against a particular facility.

- The National Center for Assisted Living and the American Health Care Association provide additional details and tips on picking an assisted-living facility at ProviderMagazine.com, the website for the organizations' monthly digest.

RESEARCH AND VISIT PROSPECTIVE FACILITIES

Once you have decided assisted living is the best option, ask your doctor or geriatric specialist for a list of appropriate local facilities, and make an appointment to visit them with your parent or relative. Bring along a checklist of things to look for and questions to ask the staff. Among them:

- Does the facility suit your relative's tastes?

- Is it clean, well-lit, and have a pleasant atmosphere?

- Are safety features — such as grab bars on all the walls and nonslip flooring materials — evident?

- How is the food quality, and is there a nutritionist on staff, are special diets accommodated, and are kosher options available?

- How does the staff interact with the residents?

- Are the administrators cheerful and respectful?

- Are residents engaged in organized activities?

- Are there enough employees to manage the residents (ask how many employees are assigned to each resident)?

- Is a licensed nurse on duty or on call at all times?

- How much training do the workers have in emergency care, first aid, and dealing with mental health issues?

You should also obtain a copy of the admissions contract and residence rules, outlining costs, services, residents' rights, and the administration of medication, special diets, and other particular residents' needs.

Make sure to visit the facility several times, on different days and at different times of the day.

CALCULATE COSTS

Once you've identified the facility you think is best, be sure to review all costs, including fees for any extra services your relative may need now or in the future, down payments, potential hospitalization charges, and the potential future rate increases. Most costs for assisted living are paid out-of-pocket.

The national average monthly rate for an assisted living unit (including room, board, and a base level of personal care) was $3,550 in 2012, up from $2,379 in 2003, according to the latest figures compiled by the MetLife Mature Market Institute. But additional services can add significantly to those costs. For instance, the average additional fee for the administration of medicine is nearly $350 more a month, according to the MetLife survey.

It's also a good idea to have an attorney review the contract before you sign it. Check the website of the National Academy of Elder Law Attorneys, at NAELA.org, for one in your area.

Top 40 Assisted-Living Companies

The following 40 companies have been named among the best assisted living chains in the nation by the National Center for Assisted Living and the American Health Care Association. Most operate multiple facilities in many states.

Americare, The Arbors at Westridge Place
Sikeston, MO
www.americareusa.net
(573) 475-4652

The Arbor Company
Atlanta, GA
www.arborcompany.com
(404) 237-4026

Atria Senior Living
Louisville, KY
www.atriaseniorliving.com

Beacon Communities
Cumming, GA
www.beaconcommunities.com
(678) 947-4423

Belmont Village Senior
Houston, TX
www.belmontvillage.com
(713) 592-9200

Benchmark Senior Living
Wellesley, MA
www.benchmarkquality.com
(781) 489-7100

Benedictine Health System
Duluth, MN
www.bhshealth.org
(800) 833-7208

Brookdale Senior Living
Brentwood, TN
www.brookdaleliving.com
(855) 444-7658

Capital Senior Living Corp.
Dallas, TX
www.capitalsenior.com
(800) 635-1232

Century Park Associates
Chattanooga, TN
www.centurypa.com
(423) 485-9405

Chelsea Senior Living
Fanwood, NJ
www.chelseaseniorliving.com
(908) 654-5200

DePaul Adult Care
Rochester, NY
www.depaul.org
(585) 426-8000

Ecumen
Shoreview, MN
www.ecumen.org
(800) 221-1507

Elmcroft Senior Living
Louisville, KY
www.elmcroft.com
(502) 753-6000

Emeritus Senior Living
Seattle, WA
www.emeritus.com
(800) 429-4828

Enlivant
Menomonee Falls, WI
www.enlivant.com
(888) 252-5001

Eskaton
Carmichal, CA
www.eskaton.org
(866) 375-2866

Evangelical Lutheran Good Samaritan Society
Sioux Falls, SD
www.good-sam.com
(866) 382-1406

Extendicare Health Services
Nekoosa, WI
www.extendicare.com
(715) 886-5353

Five Star Quality Care
Newton, MA
www.fivestarseniorliving.com
(617) 796-8387

Frontier Management
Durham, OR
www.frontiermgmt.com
(503) 443-1818

Genesis HealthCare
Kennett Square, PA
www.genesishcc.com
(866) 745-CARE

Golden Living
Plano, TX
www.goldenliving.com
(855) 494-0011

HCR ManorCare
Toledo, OH
www.hcr-manorcare.com
(419) 252-5500

Hearthstone Senior Services
Beaverton, OR
www.hearthstoneseniorliving.com
(503) 520-0911

Independent Healthcare
Georgetown, TN
www.morningpointe.com
(577) 776-4683

Integral Senior Living
Carlsbad, CA
www.islllc.com
(760) 547-7000

JEA Senior Living
Vancouver, WA
www.jeaseniorliving.com
(800) 854-9442

Juniper Communities
Bloomfield, NJ
www.junipercommunities.com
(973) 661-8300

LCS
Des Moines, IA
www.lcsnet.com
(503) 875-4500

Leisure Care
Seattle, WA
www.leisurecare.com
(800) 327-3490

Life Care Centers of America
Cleveland, TN
www.lcca.com
(423) 472-9585

Merrill Gardens
Seattle, WA
www.merrillgardens.com
(800) 509-4952

National HealthCare Corp.
Murfreesboro, TN
www.nhccare.com
(615) 890-2020

Prestige Care
Vancouver, WA
www.prestigecare.com
(800) 476-9108

Ridgeline Management
Eugene, OR
www.ridgelinemc.com
(541) 686-1119

Skilled Healthcare Group
Foothill Ranch, CA
www.skilledhealthcaregroup.com
(949) 282-5800

Sun Healthcare Group/Genesis HealthCare
Irvine, CA
www.sunh.com
(866) 745-CARE

Sunrise Senior Living
McLean, VA
www.sunriseseniorliving.com
(888) 434-4648

Trilogy Health Services
Louisville, KY
www.trilogyhs.com
(502) 412-5847

How to Choose a Nursing Home

About one in seven Americans, aged 65 and older, will require at least some nursing home care over the course of their lives, with about 3.3 million people moving into such facilities each year. For most families, picking an appropriate home for a loved one is an agonizing process, fraught with difficult choices and challenges.

Experts recommend the following strategies to select a good nursing home:

DO YOUR HOMEWORK

Check the record and background of any home you are considering for a parent or relative by visiting the website of the federal Centers for Medicare and Medicaid Services, which regulates nursing homes, and your home state's relevant inspectional services division.

VISIT MULTIPLE TIMES

It's a good idea to check a nursing home's typical operations by visiting the facility several times — on different days and at different times of the day. Take notice of the residents and staff. Are there fewer workers on Saturdays and Sundays? How are meals handled and delivered? How much interaction do the residents have with staff members? Are the residents out of their rooms and engaging with one another and with staff — or isolated?

ASK QUESTIONS ABOUT WHAT YOU SEE

A good home will employ staff members who interact well — and frequently — with the residents. Look for homes where workers address residents by name and have an evident rapport. Take notes on what you observe and ask administrators lots of questions, including:

- What do the latest inspection reports have to say about the facility's operations?

- How were any health or safety problems resolved?

- How would the home deal with specific situations — such as your mother's dementia or your father's resistance to bathing or shaving?

- How do the nurses and aides relate with residents and one another?

- What regular events are planned, such as recreational activities, music, or arts and crafts programs?

- How are conflicts resolved?

Nation's Best Nursing Homes

Picking a nursing home for a loved one can be a daunting experience. To help consumers compare facilities by cost, quality of care, and other factors, the US Centers for Medicare & Medicaid Services — the federal agency that enforces standards for the nation's 16,000 nursing homes — has created an online "Nursing Home Compare" program (Medicare.gov/nursinghomecompare/?AspxAutoDetect CookieSupport=1) that allows for searches by zip code, city, or state.

US News recently awarded a "Best Nursing Home" designation to the following nursing homes that have earned an overall rating of five stars, the agency's highest, for at least four straight quarters (Health. USNews.com/health-news.com/health-news/best-nursing-homes/ articles/2013/02/26/us-news--world-report-releases-best-nursing -homes-2013):

Alzheimer's Resource Center of Connecticut
1261 South Main Street
Plantsville, CT 06479
www.arc-ct.org/
(860) 628-9000

Avalon Nursing Home
57 Stokes Street
Warwick, RI 02889
www.avalonnhri.com/
(401) 738-1200

Bethany Skilled Nursing Facility
97 Bethany Road
Framingham, MA 01701
www.bethanyhealthcare.org/
(508) 872-6750

Catherine Kasper Home
9601 S Union Road
Donaldson, IN 46513
www.cklc.poorhandmaids.org/Catherine%20Kasper%20
Home.php
(574) 935-1742

Charles A. Dean Memorial Hospital
364 Pritham Avenue
Greenville, ME 04441
www.cadean.org/04441
(207) 695-5200

Covenant Shores Health Center
9107 Fortuna Drive
Mercer Island, WA 98040
www.covenantshores.org/skilled-nursing-seattle
(206) 268-3039

Dahl Memorial Nursing Home
215 Sandy Street
Ekalaka, MT 59324
www.dahlmemorial.com/nursinghome.html
(406) 775-8730

De La Salle Hall
810 Newman Springs Road
Lincroft, NJ 07738
www.seniorhousingnet.com/seniorliving-detail/de-la
-salle-hall-inc_810-newman-springs-rd_lincroft_nj_07738
-510968?source=web
(732) 530-9470

Duxbury House Nursing Home
298 Kings Town Way
Duxbury, MA 02332
www.welchhrg.com/memory-care-alzheimer-disease
-massachusetts/duxbury
(781) 585-2397

Elmhurst Extended Care Center
200 East Lake Street
Elmhurst, IL 60126
www.elmhurstextendedcare.org/
(630) 516-5000

Hillhaven Nursing Center
3210 Powder Mill Road
Adelphi, MD 20783
www.hillhaven.com
(301) 937-3939

Island Nursing Home
1205 Alexander Street
Honolulu, HI 96826
www.ucomparehealthcare.com/nhs/island_nursing_home/
(808) 946-5027

J Arthur Dosher Memorial Hospital
924 N Howe Street
Southport, NC 28461
www.dosher.org/getpage.php?name=index
(910) 457-3800

Jamaica Hospital Transitional Care Unit
8900 Van Wyck Expressway
Jamaica, NY 11418
www.jamaicahospital.org/pages/clinical_services/rehab/
TheTransitionalCareUnit.html
(718) 206-6595

Jeanne Jugan Residence
185 Salem Church Road
Newark, DE 19713
www.littlesistersofthepoordelaware.org
(302) 368-5886

Katahdin Nursing Home
22 Walnut Street
Millinocket, ME 04462
www.wellness.com/dir/2505477/nursing-home/me/
millinocket/katahdin-nursing-home#referrer
(207) 723-4711

Little Sisters of the Poor
1028 Benton Avenue
Pittsburgh, PA 15212
www.littlesistersofthepoorpittsburgh.org
(412) 307-1100

Lourdes Health Care Center, IN
345 Belden Hill Road
Wilton, CT 06897
www.lourdeshealth.net/
(203) 762-3318

Matulaitis Nursing Home
10 Thurber Road
Putnam, CT 06260
www.matulaitisnh.org
(860) 928-7976

Menig Extended Care
44 South Main Street
Randolph, VT 05060
www.giffordmed.org/services/menig_extended_care.shtml
(802) 728-2125

Passavant Area Hospital
1600 W Walnut Street
Jacksonville, IL 62650
www.passavanthospital.com
(217) 245-9541

Peconic Landing at Southold Inc.
1500 Brecknock Road
Greenport, NY 11944
www.peconiclanding.com
(631) 477-3800

Pioneer Lodge
300 W 3rd Street
P.O. Box 487
Coldwater, KS 67029
www.hospital-data.com/hospitals/PIONEER-LODGE-
COLDWATER.html
(620) 582-2123

Providence Seaside Hospital
725 S Wahanna Road
Seaside, OR 97138
www.oregon.providence.org/location-directory/p/providence-
seaside-hospital?utm_source=
providence-org-northcoast&utm_medium=redirect&utm_
content=providence-org-northcoast
(503) 717-7135

Quyanna Care Center
P.O. Box 966
Nome, AK 99762
www.manta.com/c/mm28ylz/quyanna-care-center
(907) 443-3311

**Rady Children's Convalescent Hospital Distinct
Part Skilled Nursing Facility**
3020 Children's Way
San Diego, CA 92123
http://health.usnews.com/best-nursing-homes/area/ca/rady
-childrens-convalescent-hospital-distinct-part-skilled-nursing
-facility-05A292
(858) 966-5833

Rehabilitation Pavilion at the Weils
16695 Chillicothe Road
Chagrin Falls, OH 44023
www.theweils.org
(440) 543-4221

Riverview Lutheran Care Center
1841 East Upriver Drive
Spokane, WA 99207
www.riverviewretirement.org
(509) 483-6483

South Mountain Restoration Center
10058 South Mountain Road
South Mountain, PA 17261
www.southmountainsanatorium.blogspot.com/
(717) 749-3121

St. Vincent Care Center
335 South Seton Avenue
Emmitsburg, Maryland 21727
www.caring.com/local/nursing-homes-in-emmitsburg-
maryland/st-vincent-care-center
(301) 447-6026

Subacute/Saratoga
13425 Sousa Lane
Saratoga, CA 95070
www.subacutesaratoga.com
(408) 378-8875

The Colony at Eden Prairie
431 Prairie Center Drive
Eden Prairie, MN 55344
www.the-colony.org
(952) 828-9500

Tockwotton on the Waterfront
500 Waterfront Drive
East Providence, RI 02914
www.tockwotton.org
(401) 272-5280

Vi at Grayhawk, a Vi and Plaza Companies Community
7501 East Thompson Peak Parkway
Scottsdale, AZ 85255
www.viliving.com/communities/scottsdale-grayhawk
(480) 361-3200

Westchester Meadows
55 Grassland Road
Valhalla, NY 10595
www.westchestermeadows.org
(914) 989-7800

Wheaton Franciscan Healthcare-Lakeshore Manor
1320 Wisconsin Avenue
Racine, WI 53403
www.mywheaton.org/locations/transitional-long-term-care/
profile/?id=13
(262) 687-2241

Wibaux County Nursing Home
712 Wibaux Street S
Wibaux, MT 59353
www.wibauxconursinghome.com
(406) 796-2429

Additional Resources for Long-Term Care

If you need further help finding long-term care for yourself or someone close to you, numerous resources are available. Among them: Medicare. Although Medicare generally doesn't pay for long-term care, the federal program offers an extensive online guide to choosing long-term care, types of services available, and comparative information on pricing and financing options, as well as links to counseling and assistance resources: Medicare.gov/what-medicare-covers/part-a/other-long-term-care-choices.html, **(800) MEDICARE, (877) 486-2048 (TTY).**

AARP: The AARP website offers a consumer's guide to long-term care options, including home care services and nursing home care: AARP.org, **(888) OUR-AARP, (877) 434-7598 (TTY).**

Aging and Disability Resource Center: The ADRC website provides information on the services offered in all 50 states, as well as Washington, DC, Guam, the Northern Mariana Islands, and Puerto Rico: ADRC-tae.acl.gov.

Care Conversations: An initiative led by the American Healthcare Association and the National Center for Assisted Living (AHCA/NCAL), this organization offers info on nursing homes, assisted living facilities, home healthcare, tips on coping with and caring for someone with Alzheimer's, and writing an advance directive: CareConversations.org, **(202) 842-4444.**

Centers for Independent Living: A state-by-state listing of CILs, which offer assistance to people with disabilities of all ages and incomes, can be found at the center's website: NCIL.org, **(877) 525-3400.**

Consumer Reports: The nation's leading, non-profit, consumer-oriented magazine offers a comprehensive analysis of long-term care insurance policies and planning tips at ConsumerReports.org.

Family Caregiver Alliance: This advocacy group offers advice and support for caregivers through its website, along with answers to commonly asked questions: Caregiver.org, **(800) 445-8106.**

The National Consumer Voice for Quality Long-Term Care: This advocacy organization provides state and local resources and consumer fact sheets with information on residents' rights and selecting a nursing home: TheConsumerVoice.org, **(202) 332-2275.**

US Department of Health and Human Service's Administration on Aging: This federal government website, AOA.gov, serves as a clearinghouse for information on long-term care, including links to state and local agencies serving older adults and their caregivers. Assistance for seniors falling under HHS' wide umbrella of services, including a wealth of data about the limitations of coverage within Medicare and resources on long-term-care insurance can be found at: ACL.gov, LongTermCare.gov, and ElderCare.gov. All entities listed here can also be reached by dialing **(800) 677-1116** or **(202) 619-0724.**

Index